Advance

Pain Free Everyday is the perfect blend of science and practical application. While myofascial release has been shown to be a very helpful treatment for fibromyalgia, access to that treatment is a challenge for many patients. *Pain Free Everyday* puts tools into the hands of those patients for self-treatment and management. Living with a chronic illness can often make one feel powerless. This book and The Fascianation Method work to give some of that power back.

–TAMI STACKELHOUSE, Founder
International Fibromyalgia Coaching Institute
IFCInstitute.com

As a defensive tactics expert who trained FBI agents, Special Forces, law enforcement officers, and Hostage Rescue Teams, I am no stranger to chronic pain. Multiple fractures, wear and tear have taken their toll. There is only so much door kicking a hip can take and both of mine need replacement. Luckily I found the Fascination Method during a retreat and Eileen Paulo-Chrisco's and Anthony Chrisco's book *Pain Free Everyday*. After reading this book, I understand why I haven't been able to change my pain without medication in the past! I'm excited to use the Fascianator to increase my mobility and to be able to fully enjoy being out and about with my seven-year old son.

–ANDREW LAWLESS, Strategic Interventionist
Author of *Blood Sugar in Check*

Roll, roll, roll your pain out of your body with The Fascianation Method! This easy read is like a mini medical journal. It provides simple self-care tips for your everyday pain. Roll out pain in a natural way...freedom.

Anthony and Eileen did a fabulous job preparing The Fascianation Method for everyone who suffers with chronic pain. It's tried, tested, and true to its purpose. Pain free naturally, with your own hands, at your own pace, in your own place. No more going to facilities for someone else to do the work.

–**PAMELA LITTLE**, Author of
It's Not Me, It's my Brain

This book causes me to feel invigorated and more curious about how to best listen and best treat my body. It even "predicts" speed bumps on the road to wellness and gives me concrete suggestions to keep on the path. I can do this! I feel more inspired and confident that I can maintain a more consistent, healthier, satisfying and generous way of living. *Pain Free Everyday* is a book I will keep close to me to refer to again and again as I recommend it to others. In Eileen's Paulo-Chrisco's words, "Reconnecting with your fascia can affect your motivation, sense of well-being and embodiment."

–**ELLA DECASTRO BARON**, Author of
Itchy Brown Girl Seeks Employment

Pain Free Everyday

Pain Free
Everyday

The Roadmap for Natural Treatment
When Pills, Injections, or Surgery
Aren't Your Solutions

EILEEN PAULO-CHRISCO
ANTHONY CHRISCO

NEW YORK

LONDON • NASHVILLE • MELBOURNE • VANCOUVER

Pain Free Everyday

The Roadmap for Natural Treatment When Pills, Injections, or Surgery Aren't Your Solutions

Published in New York, New York, by Morgan James Publishing in partnership with Difference Press. Morgan James is a trademark of Morgan James, LLC.
www.MorganJamesPublishing.com

ISBN 9781642795059 paperback
ISBN 9781642795066 eBook
ISBN 9781642795196 audio
Library of Congress Control Number: 2019902190

Cover Design by:
Christopher Kirk
www.GFSstudio.com

Interior Design by:
Chris Treccani
www.3dogcreative.net

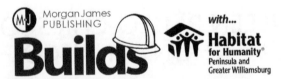

Morgan James is a proud partner of Habitat for Humanity Peninsula and Greater Williamsburg. Partners in building since 2006.

Get involved today! Visit
MorganJamesPublishing.com/giving-back

Dedication

For Channing and Malia, our motivation to stay encouraged, have faith, and never give up.

For our parents, Ed and Norma, and Michael and Huy, our favorite everyday heroes and examples of perseverance and unconditional love.

Table of Contents

Foreword

Have you ever had the feeling that something in your life was not quite right? You were feeling unfulfilled, there was creativity waiting to come from you, but there was no outlet. You felt stifled in your work. Relationships did not seem as harmonious as you knew they could be. You knew that you should be happy because you had all the tools, but the choices that you've had to make in your life did not seem to allow you to realize that happiness. That is what I've come to know as divine discontent. It is something that gives us just enough pain to make us feel that we need to be different. We need to do something more. We need to give something from inside of us that is longing to come out. This feeling oftentimes gives birth to dreams, and *dreams that are sown with the seeds of divine discontent have the greatest capacity for fruition.* We oftentimes experience this divine discontent as pain – emotional, physical, mental.

This is what I saw the author of this book, Eileen Paulo-Chrisco, going through when she came to me for pain relief. There was something waiting to come from her life and her creativity that she was longing to share with the world, but the work that she was doing wasn't taking her in the direction she needed to go. Pain is a great motivator – one of the best. And her soul's urging was not going to give up on her. This book, dear reader, is the part of the fruit of that pain. The fruit of that pain also led to the salvation of many others' pain. The program that Eileen and Anthony have created has been a breakthrough for many lives. Eileen has power packed each chapter in this book with information to help lead you to your own freedom from pain. Imagine a world where you do not have to change or edit your life to accommodate your pain. Imagine developing a practice that helps you feel strong, healthy, fruitful. You are just pages away from that. Eileen covers all aspects of chronic pain generators, and helps you find ways to reduce and eliminate their effects from your life. It's all written in simple, plain language – nothing to intimidate or make you feel like you need to go to somebody to find out more. She gives you all of the information that you need. Her heart is in each line of this book, ready to support you. Start the first chapter of *Pain Free Everyday*, the next chapter of your evolving life, and join Eileen in the mission on which her dream has taken her.

–DR. ALEXE BELLINGHAM LOWE, Doctor of Chiropractic

Author's Note

You are in the right place if you are yearning for freedom from frequent discomfort, stiffness, or numbness in your body. This book is for you if you are fighting for independence from the rusted chains of chronic pain. You know you're not alone; everyone knows someone who suffers from chronic pain. Sometimes, though, you may feel alone because your issues, although addressed, have no satisfying solution and there seems to be no resolution with the professionals who should be on your side. You fall victim to your healthcare providers, insurance companies, workers' compensation, and pharmaceutical companies.

I wrote this book because Anthony and I want to give you hope and help you overcome worry, frustration, and anxiety over your pain. Your hope is within reach today. Your hope rests on a relationship that you have to rekindle and nurture. This relationship is between you and your fascia, which is the largest organ of your body. Your fascia is an extensive body-wide tissue system that senses tension and pain and communicates sensations and messages throughout your body. Your pain is a message to pay attention. If you learn to listen to what your fascia is telling you about what's *really* going on inside of you, your fascia can be your best friend instead of your worst enemy. Let your best friend help you sense, navigate through, and process your pain so that you can dispel many of your persisting discomforts and chronic pain. In this book, we will arm you with the spark and alternative weaponry to win freedom from your chronic pain-associated battles.

You'll notice that this story goes back and forth from the voice of one person to two. That is because while I actually wrote the book, there genuinely are two hearts and two minds that allowed this self-healing roadmap to come to fruition. Without Anthony, I could not have started writing this book, or have finished it. Anthony's passion and perseverance to educate the masses about how to take care of their fascia is magnetic. Powers from above and within Anthony and me finally aligned to allow me to put our thoughts and experiences on paper.

Introduction

"There is a voice that doesn't use words. Listen."
– Rumi

When I'm in the canoe in the middle of the ocean, I feel free. My senses are aware. Smelling and tasting the sea mist, hearing the wind, feeling the buoyancy and the power of the waves is exhilarating. I feel fortunate to be surrounded by the beautiful mountains, textured clouds, the vast sky, huge sea turtles, schools of fish, and the light refracting in the water. I look forward to being amongst the dolphins and relish the sound of swishing and crashing water on the canoe. I'm a tiny part of a vast universe. I feel God; I feel alive and in touch with my soul. Though there are challenges in my life, though there's a list of chores and things to do, they don't get to take a ride with me in the canoe. They aren't hovering around me either. Being in the middle of the ocean is my sanctuary that's devoid of clutter – physical and mental. I'm at peace and exhilarated at the same time.

I enjoy ocean paddling because I feel empowered. I feel grateful. The only things I judge are my decisions on how to act and react to the wind, to the current, to the experienced or novice kayaker or boat that is coming my way, and to the guidance of my teammates. I usually paddle in a six-woman canoe, an OC-6. There's a vibration that each of us in the canoe share. When our vibrations are in sync, we glide above the water with ease. When we aren't in sync, when imbalances exist that aren't quickly corrected, the canoe rocks, there's more drag, and there can be a ripple effect of lost momentum.

In a race, we truly want to win. In a competition, fear and panic do not serve us. They can put us into a feedback loop of negative energy and the ability to stay on point with the tasks at hand and to strive for the goal is hampered. When I have negativity, fear, or panic, I take advice from Deepak Chopra: STOP

S = Stop
T = Take deep breaths
O =Observe
P = Proceed with kindness, joy, and love (for what you are doing and for those around you)

After taking a few seconds to STOP, we forge forward and keep our eye on the prize. We win some, we lose some, but we gain more experience, wisdom, and pleasure!

One day my loving husband, Anthony, blessed me with my own one-person canoe, an OC-1. After the purchase, it was months before I could get it out on the water. I first needed to find transportation, at least a rack to transport the canoe. Finally, we had a truck, a rack, and the OC-1 in our backyard ready to go. One random grey-skied morning, Anthony insisted that we have no excuses, and we were going to get me into the canoe on actual flowing water. Anthony was so determined with good intent that I couldn't say no. I knew I wasn't ready. I had never paddled in an OC-1 and never used a foot pedal for steering, but we packed the canoe onto my son's truck and headed to Haleiwa for my first voyage!

I hopped in the canoe, paddled a few yards forward, and huli'd. "Huli" is capsizing in an outrigger canoe. I got back in, paddled around to my heart's content, and let my son give it a go. I watched his technique from shore. He huli'd as well, then paddled quite a way out. After my son came back in, I was initially content not to go in again because I didn't have a paddling buddy. The kayak rental next to us had run out of kayaks. Oh well, I thought. I'd go for a super quick paddle to get a better feel for the OC-1. My son found the canoe leash awkward, so I decided that I wouldn't wear the canoe leash. I'm not a strong swimmer, but I wasn't going very far out anyway. The further I paddled out without huli'ing, the further I wanted to paddle. I was shooting for a buoy about a half mile from shore. When I got near the buoy, more cloud coverage started creeping in, and I remembered that I wasn't properly fueled. Heading back to shore, I huli'd.

The water was cooler. Where I was, the water was pretty deep, but I was lucky to stumble onto an underwater rock, which seemed very random. I was able to stand and flip my canoe right-side-up. I got back in the boat, had my eye on the shoreline prize, resumed paddling, but no prize yet – I was heading back down underwater again. Another huli. I was loving myself. Though I did not plan well (I didn't plan *at all*), I set myself up for this challenge. I couldn't put myself into the negative self-talk, energy-sapping ego/mind game.

My spirit was speaking with God. My spirit kept my mind above water, afloat. I was determined to get back into the canoe, figure out how to paddle back in without capsizing. Mind over matter. I had paddling experience (albeit with at least four other ladies in a six-man canoe). I just had to keep my canoe at the correct angle, keep paddling, and figure out what strength of my strokes and positioning and angling of my torso would keep my canoe upright and get me back to land, where my dog and my son awaited. Easy! I'd figure out patterns and I'd make the proper corrections. Well, the wind started kicking up. All of a sudden, I found myself underwater with a canoe to flip over. While holding on to my paddle, I flipped the canoe right-side-up and hoisted myself back in the boat with even more determination. Shoot, I realized that I had to make a U-turn. I should have flipped my canoe to face the shore before I got back in. I also noticed that the current took me further away from my destination. I had to figure out the maneuvering quickly. It was getting windier and starting to sprinkle. *C'mon Eileen, paddle up!* I made a successful U-turn and paddled further in, and as soon as I began mentally celebrating my first U-turn in a windy situation, I was back down in the water. I decided that it was easier for me to hang on to my canoe and paddle and swim to shore. I didn't have the energy to undergo another huli.

Every fifty strokes I took a break to assess my successes. The good news was that I was making headway and the sprinkling had stopped. The bad news was that my nose was bleeding. I have a hereditary blood vessel condition called hereditary hemorrhagic telangiectasia, so I'm always prepared for a nosebleed. Yes, even in the middle of the ocean. I shoved a wad of Kleenex up my bleeding nostril. Thank God both nostrils weren't bleeding. For a quick second, I thought about sharks. People say that chances of getting bit by a shark are slim, *but* if you play in the Hawaiian waters, chances are greater. In fact, while swimming on the other side of the island, my former boss had a real battle with a shark. After a lengthy battle and finally gauging the shark's eye out, my boss won the battle but lost his leg to amputation. That was very close to home. Luckily, in the thick of survival mode (I *had* to get back to my family), my thoughts quickly returned to counting another fifty strokes forward.

Next assessment, the current pushed my progress back out and I looked forward to an energy-expending swim ahead of me. I had to rest. My breakfast of champions, half of a Cliff bar, must have burned off. My hat was falling off my head because the Velcro strap somehow ripped off. As I readjusted my hat, I heard a Godsend. His name was Leonard. He paddled over to me in his OC-1 and asked if I was all right. I confessed that I was stuck and had been warned not to take the canoe out when windy. Leonard agreed: it was too windy for me to be out paddling; the winds were twenty-five to thirty mph. Without judgment, he advised me to check the wind report next time. With Leonard's much need guidance and moral support, I decided to try paddling to a jetty nearby instead of shooting for the shore. I jumped back into the canoe, paddled only a few yards over, and torqued back into the beautiful waters of the North Shore, Hawaii. This time, with someone by my side.

Something didn't feel right. Besides ill preparation, I just couldn't figure out why I couldn't stay in the boat. I flipped the boat over again to jump back in the saddle. The next thing I saw, my canoe was downwind from me and my paddle was... somewhere. My brain went into *what in tarnation* mode. I didn't have time for that! Leonard held my boat and yelled, "Swim, swim!" Swimming, counting five strokes at a time, I felt I was approaching my canoe. I had to approach my canoe! "You have to paddle harder! C'mon, *harder!*" Out loud, I proclaimed "C'mon Eileen. You can do this!" I got close enough to grab onto my canoe leash (which later I learned that I definitely should have strapped on when I flipped my boat upright), pulled the canoe to me, and caught my breath. I knew the drill. I flipped my OC-1 right-side-up. "Where's your paddle? You have to get your paddle!" Leonard exclaimed. Swallowing my pride, I admitted that I didn't have the energy to swim for my paddle. Leonard got the cue and retrieved my paddle, allowing me to catch my breath and take off my dang ill-fitting all-purpose water/yoga/airplane rubber bottomed socks, which caused a lot of drag. The water was too choppy for me to be towed in by hanging onto Leonard's canoe, so Leonard flagged a lifeguard from the beach that we were drifting toward.

The lifeguard came and we swapped our watercrafts. I was instructed to take the lifeguard's surfboard and paddle along the shoreline, then into the shore of the beach next to my original destination. Leonard decided to paddle behind me, encouraging me to keep paddling, paddle harder, change up my strokes for better efficiency. I was so encouraged because I was sent another lifeline, but *I was spent!* I was running on less oxygen with one obstructed nostril. Much safer now on top of a monstrosity of a lifeguard longboard, I had time to think. Think about how silly it was for me to go out paddling without doing my homework: researching OC-1 techniques, checking the wind, checking the equipment, drinking plenty of water, eating a real breakfast, etc.

"Paddle harder! You have to keep your left arm down in the water to veer inland and paddle strong with your right arm!" I didn't agree with the paddling advice, but I couldn't let the negativity set in. I couldn't let my thoughts interfere with the prize of finally reaching land. Listen to the waterman, Eileen. He knows what he's talking about. I kept paddling and even reverted to my two-arm paddling style, which gave me more power.

"Don't paddle with your left arm! Put your left arm in the water and paddle with your right! Stronger!" This went on and on for minutes, and a new lifeguard emerged from the shore. "You have to paddle stronger," was coming in stereo. But the lifeguard was yelling for me to paddle with both arms and head for the shore. "What are you doing?" he frustratingly kept yelling. I was confused, tired, but just like Dory, just kept swimming, just kept swimming. The volley of conflicting commands continued and finally, as the current and wind died down, the lifeguard swam out to me, hopped onto the surfboard, and paddled us back in to shore. When I got back to shore, I learned from Lifeguard #1 that the rudder of my OC-1 didn't work. The rudder wire was disconnected from the foot pedal.

This happened for a reason. It was more than a lesson in proper preparation and planning. It was a lesson in exercising my voice. I could have said no to trying out the OC-1 that day, knowing I hadn't done my research, but I hadn't wanted to let anyone down. It was a lesson in not giving up, staying focused to stay on task. It was a lesson in staying positive and having faith. I had the right tools, and though I lacked a lot of wisdom, every minute of positivity and determination, reinforcement, and faith granted me time and more energy for better things to happen. I had three godsends: Leonard, Lifeguard #1, and Lifeguard #2. They steered me away from fear and panic. I was thankful that my nosebleed was contained, because some days, I swear I lose a pint of blood. Though it wasn't really treacherous out there, I really could have had a bad outcome. I was meant to come back intact and with more purpose.

I know that I was put on this Earth for great things. Before my ninety-eight-year old grandmother passed away, she summoned me to travel to the Philippines so that she could pass down her "power" – her "Anting Anting," which symbolizes healing power – to me before she died. She wanted to die but she believed that God wouldn't take her until she passed down her power. Months after I visited, my grandmother passed. She was a midwife, although she never studied midwifery in school. Perhaps the power that I acquired is the power to help women "give birth" to new joy, a new life. Rebirth.

I know that one of these great things I was destined for is to finally share the contents of this book. So many women suffer from chronic pain. We are nurturers, and often while nurturing others, we neglect ourselves. When we neglect ourselves long enough, we may lose our spirit and some joy. I hope you take the information in this book and take action with a real solution, our fascial-care program for your pain. Your fascia is like a computer hard drive because it stores and retrieves information, even information about the computer's operating system. If your hard drive is maintained and operating smoothly, your machine will function efficiently. If your hard drive is full and/or infected by a virus, malware, or physical damage, your computer will slow down, get sick, and, if left unaddressed, terminate all programs. Now is the time to reboot your proverbial hard drive before your body succumbs to adrenal burnout, depression, other dysfunction, or chronic illness. Rebalance and realign without pills, without surgery, without doubt. Now join Anthony and me while we take you on a journey through the amazing world of fascia!

Chapter 1:

Don't Stop Believing

"When you have exhausted all possibilities,
remember this - you haven't."
– Thomas Edison

Jeannette: Fifty-six, hairdresser, always taken sports seriously but after years of working, road running, biking, and swimming, she developed sciatica; neck, shoulder, and postural issues; arthritis in her fingers; and even a small bone spur on her hand from scissor overuse. She envisioned not being able to work if she didn't find a solution for her pain.

Mindy: Fifty-year-old who used to be an athlete and pushed her body to the limits in her younger years. She endured years of hand and shoulder pain, tingling, and numbness of her limbs. All her joints became frozen; she was diagnosed with carpal tunnel syndrome and wasn't able to perform at work due to her pain and mobility restrictions.

She was getting depressed and withdrawn. She took over-the-counter pain medications but didn't want to take medication to camouflage the pain for the rest of her life.

Val: Fifty-two, stuck behind a desk, computer, or the wheel of her car most days. She suffered from allergies for as long as she could remember, and had feet and arch pain, sore creaking knees, sciatic pain, headaches, carpal tunnel syndrome, and fibromyalgia. Exercising for ten minutes on an elliptical trainer kept her in pain for days. She was in so much chronic pain that she lost quality time with her family. Her husband could not even touch her. After an increase in blood pressure from taking so many medications, Val was beginning to accept that it was only downhill from here. Her pains, her body falling apart, and the pharmaceuticals she relied on seemed just an inevitable part of getting older.

Char: Sixty-two, a retired teacher who swam miles multiple times a week and led a very active, athletic lifestyle until her injuries led to limited mobility of her shoulder, pain in her neck, and bilateral knee replacements. Post-surgery she developed IT band syndrome, her knees continued to be problematic, and she tore a calf muscle in physical therapy.

Grace: Late thirties, a traveling medical doctor who enjoyed yoga, hiking, biking, and surfing. After a work relocation that involved hours of driving, she had a new stiffness in her back. Circumstances prevented her from attending yoga classes, and her back stiffness became quite painful. She worked through the pain. She didn't believe in taking medications for back pain and saw far too many patients become addicted to medications and have terrible side effects.

Fran: Fifty-six, a very active self-employed fitness coach. She spent two years doing expensive and painful therapy to regain mobility from painful frozen shoulder, but the pain sometimes persisted. She developed frozen shoulder in her other shoulder and couldn't lift her arm above her head without excruciating pain. Bumping into anything caused pain. She worried about how she'd be able to work with arms that weren't working correctly. She wondered where to find someone to help her heal without feeling like her arm was breaking in the process. There was no way she'd go through surgery to get her shoulder "fixed."

Do any of these stories resonate with you or someone you know? In 2016 the Center for Disease Control estimated that about fifteen million people live with severe joint pain or discomfort. If you've ever suffered from joint pain, you know how life-altering the pain can be. Things that we all take for granted like getting dressed, brushing our hair, driving, doing household chores, and bringing in the groceries take more time. Bathing, holding a coffee mug, or sitting still can be frightening. You may have sleepless nights of concern and discomfort, leading to lethargy, moodiness, and fogginess. You may withdraw from relationships and feel defeated, even depressed. The things you identified yourself with being – a hard-worker, an involved parent or grandparent, a dynamic team member, a creative artist, or an independent person – can suddenly be taken away. When you lose the ability to do the things that you love, you may find new things to enjoy but still feel a void. Is this void eroding your soul?

You may not even want to admit that your joint pain is chronic pain. You call it discomfort because chronic pain would interfere with your heroic multitasking ability or beast mode workout. After some rest, stretching, and analgesics, you push through the discomfort, and you're able to resume your normal routine. Once the annoyance comes back again, you subconsciously engage different muscles. You strategize by modifying your technique or lightening your purse load, but next thing you know your swagger has changed. You walk differently although your shoes are the same, you switch to a smaller purse, and your resting facial expression is peculiar. It's not quite resting witch face, but rather uneasy, concerned woman face.

This progression of disuse and dysfunction is common. You are not alone. Look around when you're at church, at your kid's sports games, standing in line at the grocery store, or walking around the gym. Do you notice people rubbing their necks, pressing between their necks and shoulders, cradling their elbows, nonchalantly digging their thumbs into their lower backs or hips? These gestures of discomfort typically precede the donning of band-aids of many forms: compression sleeves, wrapped bandages, boots, braces, shoe inserts, therapy tape, and even magnetic therapy jewelry.

These band-aids may alleviate your joint pain but don't address the root of it. They immobilize the joint and minimize inflammation, but when the root cause of joint pain isn't addressed, the problem will move up or down the chain to other parts of your body. One day you have shoulder pain, then months later, without any accidents or known injury, you may have thumb pain. Unresolved pain and grief can lead to all kinds of "shuns" – dysfunc"shun," prescript"shuns," addict"shun," or depress"shun," which we all want to shun – reject. The pain becomes dysfunction. Use of aspirin, ibuprofen, naproxen, or narcotics masks the pain while silently causing other damage to organs and often leads to addiction. It's known that depression and pain share some of the same nerve pathways, so depression is often a downstream result of chronic pain. Add the imbalance of age-related or stress-induced hormonal shifts, and it's no wonder that by mid-life, even the strongest of human minds and bodies perceive pain, dis-ease, and crisis.

If you're like Jeanette, Mindy, Val, Char, Grace, or Fran, you do not want to resort to surgical intervention, and you do not want to rely on taking pills daily to manage your pain. You don't want to resign to the "fact" that you'll have to live with your joint pain forever.

Read on to learn how The Fascianator® and The Fascianation Method®, a natural self-care method that Anthony and I developed, brought back freedom from pain for these real-life women. We hope that you take the time to read here and now what we love sharing with others. Like thousands of women have already experienced, you are stumbling upon revolutionary information to empower yourself and tap into your ability to self-heal and maintain mind-body balance.

Believe in your capacity, stay committed to yourself, and you too can be happier, filled with more joy, and enjoy pain free living in your prime and beyond!

Jeanette: "I'm on zero medication and say the same thing directly after my early-morning roller session: I feel lighter, brighter, energized, and above all, pain free. So I cannot recommend The Fascianator enough. The only thing that really amazes me is that if it takes just one hour of our day to feel this good, why aren't we all doing it?"

Mindy: "It has been two years since I was taught about how to care for my fascia, and The Fascianation Method has eliminated that pain I was waking to each morning. I roll four times a week and have eliminated the surgery option the doctor recommended. I very rarely take pain medication, and I feel like I did in my twenties. I recommend everyone give it a try. The Fascianation Method has given me a new life!"

Val: "I am no longer on any medication. I am pain free. I have never felt this good, probably not for the last fifteen to twenty years. My husband said, 'I have my wife back.' You know, many times people just give up way too soon and you just need to go through the process. No pain, no gain, but it works."

Char: "I feel (the) self-myofascial release program has been extremely beneficial…I practice two to three days a week. The pain and discomfort caused by my IT band is no longer present. The flexibility and range of motion in my knees have improved dramatically (I can now do a complete squat), and I am now walking up and down stairs with ease. I am able to swim one or more miles without pain or discomfort, four to five times per week. The Fascianation Method changed my entire life."

Grace: "I was willing to try anything. I was practicing yoga and I felt better than I had when the pain first started. However, I wanted to be back to where I was before I ever had any pain! I bought a Fascianator and took a private lesson to learn how to use it. I am so glad that I did not resort to taking painkillers or surgery for my back pain. I have seen too many patients do these things. Unfortunately, their pain often recurs even after surgery, or they become dependent on medications. But I know how to ameliorate my pain when I have it. It is empowering."

Fran: "The Fascianation Method has given me freedom to live again! I no longer feel helpless. I feel empowered that I can take care of my own body and that aging does not have to include aches and pains that won't go away. I believe in The Fascianation Method so much that I became an instructor myself, and now it is my absolute joy to help others relieve their aches and pains themselves."

Chapter 2:
Our Story

*"The miracle is this – the more we share
the more we have."*
– Leonard Nimoy

What are the chances that my fourth-grade classmate, a boy who had a crush on me since we were twelve and who I ignored all the way through high school, ended up being my husband and business partner with the mission to change lives – many lives? Neither Anthony nor I could have predicted that our personal and professional fates would converge to create a pioneering process and a self-massage tool that would change thousands of lives!

I've been blessed and cursed with unique learning opportunities that came together in ways I didn't expect. The universe guided me through astonishing highs and lows, which gave me amazing insight into chronic pain relief that I've been destined to share with you. I am not a doctor, nor a physical therapist. Rather, I am a founding member of the Fascia Research Society, one of only 263 founding members in the world. I've spent almost two decades as a scientific researcher whose work has contributed to the research of 2009 Nobel Laureate for Physiology or Medicine, Dr. Elizabeth Blackburn. I'm also an entrepreneur, certified personal trainer, group fitness instructor, information age wife, and mother. Probably like you, I've endured decades of business and busy-ness that have led to my own chronic pain woes.

My destiny was to share my journey side-by-side with Anthony. Anthony has been in the post-rehabilitation business for almost twenty-five years. Collectively, Anthony and I have dedicated over forty-five years to learning about what happens to the body when it is imbalanced. We've both had our fair share of annoyances and joint pain that have riddled us for decades. Together, our passions have led to discovering what many other professionals with more formal education and more professional practice constraints (protocols, healthcare system) have yet to figure out. We've learned how to create the neutrality of the body so that the body can do what it was designed to do: heal itself. We co-developed a chronic pain relief program, The Fascianation Method for self-care that realigns, restores, resets, and revitalizes the body. Actually, the method was Anthony's brainchild, and I offered scientific discussion and support over the years. The program focuses on self-care of the body's soft tissues, which can be the root cause of havoc in the body.

When I was in grade school, I knew that I wanted to be a medical doctor. I wanted to help people relieve their physical and psychological discomforts from ailments. I was a relatively healthy kid but suffered from allergies, bad eczema, and other painful and embarrassing skin issues that other kids wondered and joked about. I hated being poked and prodded as a specimen at the doctor's office. I hated taking the daily red pill that sapped my energy. I hated wearing long sleeves and pants in the summer to hide my red, flaky skin. Having to switch creams and ointments every few months was such a drag. The biggest drag was being unable to play with the intensity that other kids did because I was a tomboy at heart. The lethargy, the sting of my face, and the cracking skin in the folds of my joints was such a buzzkill.

During those awkward years, I met Anthony. In the fourth grade, we lived in different parts of town and were bussed to the same school. We were thrown into the town's "Mentally Gifted Minors" program, where inattentive, hyper, quirky, and quickly bored kids united in a new school. That year I wrote my first term paper, entitled *The Biology of the Cell*. We were misunderstood kids with offbeat interests and intensities. Although segregated from the other students, who teased or bullied many of us, we thrived in our new community of shared geekiness, creativity, and intellect. Anthony and I were hardly the best of buddies. Anthony, having occasional classroom outbursts, kicked a kickball smack dab into my stomach and stomped on my foot running into second base. He sometimes seemed like a punk. I recall punching him in the hallway and being teased that I punched him because I liked him. Perhaps to prove people wrong, I ignored him. I was a tenacious kid. I ignored him in junior high, ignored him in high school band, and even ignored him in my own house when Anthony came over for baritone practice with my brother. It wasn't until I bumped into him after college that I finally gave a second thought to friendship with Anthony.

After college, to buy time to get into medical school, I landed a research technician job at The Geraldine Brush Cancer Research Institute, under the directorship of professor Helene Smith, cytogeneticist, pioneering breast cancer researcher, and chairwoman of the oversight committee for the Department of Defense's $200 million grant programs for cancer research. I was so fortunate to be in the company of talented teams with phenomenal mentors, collaborations, and resources. Complementary medicine therapies, as well as Western medicine approaches, were being explored. There I even met Yeshi Dhonden, a traditional Tibetan practitioner who was the Dalai Lama's 20-year personal physician. Suffering from a relapse of breast cancer, Helene was passionate about exploring Tibetan low-tech avenues that Western medicine's one-size-fits-all diagnoses and therapies lack. The open exchange of knowledge and passion could bridge the gap between traditional Eastern medicine and Western medicine.

My primary role at the lab was to isolate cellular and tissue material from clinical samples for laboratory examination and research. I learned the art of tissue culture, meticulously cultivating, propagating, and manipulating breast cells in dishes or flasks. My cultures were like my babies. They were to be treated with respect since they were once living tissue in someone, who cared to donate their tissue for research. On a regular schedule, whether a work day, sick day or holiday, I stared at and nurtured my cells, looking for changes in and around them. I fed my cells with fresh food, quality food, removed the waste products that surrounded them, made sure the cells had enough space to grow and air to breathe but weren't too isolated from their neighbors. Cells are like people. They have nutrient needs, communication needs, waste removal needs, and spatial needs. I learned how to tweak the cells' environmental conditions to alter the cells' behavior and gene expression. Environment plays such a massive role in happiness and health. In a poor, imbalanced environment, like cells in the lab, humans can go through stress, crisis, loss of faculties, and transformation. Sometimes I could nurture cells to recover from crisis and sometimes the cells were pushed beyond their limit to irreversible health. In the lab, I was able to chemically transform happy, genetically nonmalignant cells to become cancerous cells.

I was passionate about cells and hungry to learn as much as I could. My boss had seen no other twenty-something with bright-eyed zeal like mine for learning and working at the lab bench. My workdays were often twelve hours of repetitive motion, including weekends and holidays, either hunched over a microscope or lab equipment in a sustained poor ergonomic position. To counterbalance being cooped up in the lab all day, I'd go for a run up and down the hills of San Francisco or go to the gym after work. Lo and behold, at the gym, I ran into Anthony, my skinny old classmate who became a confident personal trainer with quite a physique and a penchant for bragging about his knowledge of the human body and movement. While Anthony showed off his bench press skills, I had a plan to show off my lab-benching skills.

One Sunday, having literal buckets of work to process, I put Anthony to work scraping off fat and cutting skin from breast reductions so that I could isolate different cell types to use for experiments. My cells were tools to investigate early molecular and genetic changes underlying the progression of breast cancer. Little did Anthony or I know at the time that we were dealing with fascia!

In the next few years our friendship blossomed. Anthony and I shared our passions for science, the human body, music, running, hiking, dancing, skiing…we were on top of the world and falling in love. Eventually we got married.

Loving life and a new career move to pharmaceutical research, I did not pursue medical school. Anthony built his career as a post-rehabilitation specialist. Do you know anyone who has had six weeks of physical therapy but isn't ready to walk up a flight of steps on her own? Or anyone whose condition became worse after physical therapy? Even after weeks of physical therapy sessions many patients have lasting symptoms and limitations, or even new problems. Anthony was phenomenal at creating and teaching exercise programs and building peoples' motivation to heal. Early in his career, he had given many people new hope, new motivation, and new opportunities. Anthony was changing new lives weekly. Under the tutelage of his favorite mentor, Erich Jenkins, Anthony quickly rose to manage, teach, and inspire other trainers in how to run a business to change lives. One thing Erich taught Anthony was, "the first day you think you know it all is the first day you're an idiot." Inspired by Anthony's healing successes, I still worked in the lab, but I also became a certified personal trainer with an emphasis in corrective exercise.

Life was great, we felt well-balanced until one day Erich Jenkins tragically died in an accident. Anthony was devastated. Not too long after Erich passed, Anthony's mother, who seemed active and healthy enough to enjoy her recent retirement, came back from a doctor's visit with a diagnosis of gas. Anthony's mother felt that her problem was more than just gas. She told her doctor that she just didn't feel right in her abdominal area. She was given Xantac to alleviate her abdominal bloating, or what the doctor referred to as her "fat stomach." There was not much dialogue and informational exchange about lifestyle or other aspects of Anthony's mother's health, such as her high blood pressure and her suboptimal thyroid hormone levels. It seemed as if the physician had one eye on the clock, one eye on the patient, and neither eye on Anthony's mom's medical record. A couple of weeks later, Anthony's mother was diagnosed with late stage ovarian cancer. After numerous surgeries, a few rounds of chemotherapy, and the last resort treatment of naturopathic tea therapy, she died within sixteen months of diagnosis at the young age of fifty-two. My mother-in-law never got to meet our kids. Understandingly, Anthony had a bitterness toward doctors and the Western medical system that he couldn't hide or shake. He felt that MDs didn't know everything, yet they operated as if they did. They operated as idiots on autopilot. At least the ones who willingly subscribed to failing medical tenets and were costing people quality of life or their lives were shameless and insensitive imbeciles.

It's unfortunate that many patients believe that their doctors are equipped with everything they need to know in order to send patients on the path of healing. Sometimes doctors don't go out of their way to try to seek more information to help their patients. Doctors may not have the time to confer with their colleagues. Patients don't go out of their way to offer more information to help their doctors. People aren't aware that they don't know enough to make sound decisions. Doctors are people. Many make conclusions on quick hunches based upon their limited training from medical school or lack of sufficient continuing education. The best they can do is merely treat the symptoms and hope the disease or ailment improves with time. This is the state of our healthcare system. To dull the pain, Anthony played a lot of video games and smoked a lot of weed.

Anthony's religious zeal for studying fascia began about five years after his mother's unfortunate death. In hindsight, having the current knowledge that we have now about stress, inflammation, sugary drinks, the dangers of a sedentary lifestyle, and fascia, he believed that he could have saved his mother from dying so young. Because he didn't take action while his mother was sick, he is taking action now. In every woman who suffers from chronic pain or chronic illness in her forties, fifties, sixties, and seventies, he sees his mother. In honor of his mother, a day has not gone by where Anthony has encouraged a woman to take the time for self-care before tending to every chore that "needs" to be completed.

Eighteen years of lab work began affecting my neck and shoulders. A poor dumbbell overhead press led to a nagging shoulder injury. Excessive sitting at work coupled with dynamic Tae Kwon Do kicks and poor stretching contributed to a few memorable episodes of debilitating back spasms. A skiing fall and a snowboarder planting his landing on my head resulted in whiplash injuries. After having my second child I developed DeQuervain's tendonitis, aka Mommy's wrist. It hurt to hang on to books, my lab tools, dumbbells, handlebars, steering wheels, dog leashes, and the baby's bottle. Joint pain sucked, but I pushed through because I couldn't stop working. I couldn't stop feeding and holding my kids. I couldn't stop walking my dogs. I was also an endorphin and movement junkie. I didn't feel complete if I didn't get my workouts in, barrel down hills skiing or riding my mountain bike, walk my dogs, or go for a run. It's funny how our pursuit for a balanced life can eventually render us imbalanced.

Anthony and I trained hard because that was what fitness trainers did, but some of our occasional aches and discomforts came with higher frequency. I laugh looking back at photos from those days because we were gym rats and winning running races, but were often adorned with wraps, straps, braces, analgesic pads, and athletic tape. Back then, we didn't believe that we had chronic pain conditions. We even moved to Hawaii so that we could live an active lifestyle with our kids and to be able to frolic outdoors 365 days a year. The move would also be a way to physically reconnect with Anthony's mother, whose ashes were spread in the ocean just off of Lanikai Beach.

Paradise was calling us! I left my previous job as an Associate Scientist and accepted a new position as a cell biologist, paid forty percent of my last salary. The lifestyle gain raising our family in sunny Hawaii would be worth the monetary loss. I was hired at a small biomedical research startup company and split my time between two bosses to support two totally different cell-based projects. Exciting! The startup had many fewer resources than I was used to having access to. That was quite challenging because the materials required for biological experiments were very costly and shipping to Hawaii was exorbitant. Early on, my motivation declined. My problem wasn't the resources, it was the support. One boss supported me very well. The other boss told me that I wasn't hired to think, I was hired to do. I was told that my job was to do only one thing. I was told that people with my education couldn't possibly read academic journal articles, plan experiments, and have the lab bench skills that I claimed I had. I was not used to a work environment in which people did not believe in my capacity. At my previous company, I won performance awards and bonuses, was encouraged to cross train in different departments, and was often left to run the lab for extended periods of time when my boss traveled abroad. Paradoxically, the experiments I designed were the same experiments that my doubtful boss developed for me to execute. Ironically, two years later, this boss was eventually let go and I was left to spearhead the cell and tissue-based effort in developing a bioengineered implant for human transplantation. My M.O. became ego-driven versus soul-driven.

It took about six years for Anthony to fine tune The Fascianation Method of self-myofascial release, our method of self-care. Previously, we each used foam rollers instead of knee wraps to heal our chronic knee pain. Foam rolling involved using cylindrical foam to roll out/self-massage for athletic conditioning. As personal trainers, we learned limited foam rolling techniques to lengthen our muscles before and after workouts. Anthony took the idea of foam rolling to treat his clients' aches and pains. Anthony was influenced by the work of John Barnes, a fifty-year physical therapist who healed peoples' chronic pain and ailments that had failed to respond to conventional therapies, medications, and surgery. As many people as Barnes healed, it seemed he had as many naysayers because soft tissue care and improving lymphatic flow weren't typical treatment strategies for common ailments. Anthony used Barnes' bodywork principles and techniques to figure out how to apply those techniques to himself. Instead of using foam rollers, he taught a class using cardboard cylinders, which were more firm and had a smaller diameter than the foam rollers of the time. I remember Anthony having all night neuroses with his collection of fascia research papers and his rigid roller prototype. I remember his excitement when he finally discovered the technique to cure his tennis elbow. Anthony hadn't even been able to close the shower curtain because his elbow hurt so severely. One night, while experimenting with various rolling positions, Anthony placed enough pressure on a particular part of his forearm to elicit a twenty second shriek. Two and a half years of suffering were alleviated in a few seconds of rolling.

Anthony taught his clients how to roll the feet, neck, forearms, and other parts people weren't rolling. Routinely on Friday nights, he had fifty people waiting in line out the door to take his rolling class. As time went by, people felt miraculous – some no longer suffered from plantar fasciitis, one woman's hypermobility syndrome was no longer problematic. Not only did people's joint pains disappear, but their constipation, migraine headaches, and ovarian cyst issues resolved. "*What is this?*" people asked Anthony. Anthony didn't have a name for his unique rolling sequence, he didn't exactly know what physiological and molecular changes were going on with these people, but he knew that his process of self-myofascial release was changing lives.

While Anthony was rolling peoples' pain away, I investigated the interactions between collagen and wound healing in lab dishes and in animal studies. When conditions around a wounded area weren't optimal, the imbalances tipped the healing response to a heightened inflammatory response. I observed that stiff and thickened tissue disrupted connections required for communication throughout the environment. I realized that unwinding stiff tissue bettered connections and communication. We can all imagine challenges arising from persisting heightened stress, poor or no communication in a work environment. Things get done improperly, inadequately, or sometimes not at all! After almost two years of very meticulously observing microenvironments, my gut told me that my collective observations throughout my years of research could explain the environmental shifts, tissue remodeling, and healing that was happening when Anthony's clients rolled. Routine rolling on the rigid roller was like stripping off the patina for an object needing restoration. The stripping allowed new connections to be established. Sharing this revelation with Anthony was the saving grace to bring back my soul.

Despite our success stories of changing lives, people still scoffed at what we felt so passionately about. Anthony and I were like broken records on repeat. People called

Anthony and his roller obsession wacko. Anthony's boss wanted to see him doing less rolling (a.k.a. healing) and more ungratifying work. People couldn't believe that I planned on leaving my stable lab job to become a full-time personal trainer. It was a blow to our enthusiasm and confidence, and there began the downward spiral. Anthony had never really processed and healed from his mother's death. I didn't understand many of his behaviors stemming from his pain, imbalance, frustration, and work dissatisfaction. His punkish attitude resurfaced. I had my own work dissatisfaction and was obsessed with trying to control things that were beyond my control. I should have been using that energy to better focus on my children. Instead of engaging in the endorphin releasing physical activity we once loved, Anthony and I turned to destructive coping patterns. We partied like it was 1999. We turned to temporary solutions that anesthetized our emotional pain. "Everything in moderation, even moderation" was our weekend motto.

Workplace stagnation, home frustrations, and imbalance caught up with me. My vigor and motivation waned; I was irritable, foggy, and anxiety ridden. I never suffered a tragic loss, but I was deeply hurt. I became deeply lost. I never seemed satisfied. It had been a while since I felt spiritually aligned. I bit the bullet and saw a psychiatrist who diagnosed me with ADHD, anxiety, and depression and prescribed me a triad of pill therapy, which exacerbated my neck, upper back, and shoulder pain. After a year of trying different anxiety and depression medicines listed on the drop-down menu for mental health treatments, I quit cold turkey. I know you're not supposed to do that for psycho-associated drugs, but besides unwanted side effects, I never felt the drugs' intended effects. I had recurring dreams that either I was in trouble being accosted or a loved one was in trouble. In my dreams, I tried to scream for help or attention, but my scream was silent or my voice was always muffled. No one was covering my mouth. I felt that someone was sitting on my chest preventing me from yelling or budging, but visually in my dream no one was holding me down.

I developed uterine polyps, my allergies that I hadn't suffered from since college resurfaced, and breast exams showed concerning tissue density changes. These changes warranted a 3D mammogram, which concerned me since I just had a dose of radiation from my routine mammogram. My frequent nosebleeds (later diagnosed as a hereditary hemorrhagic condition) started. In retrospect, I saw that I created the havoc of my internal chemistry with my thoughts and beliefs. My negative thought patterns about my work situation and my lifestyle made me chronically inflamed and sick.

Anthony fine-tuned The Fascianation Method in 2011. Due to a relatively inactive lifestyle, my chronic neck, upper back, and shoulder pains were enough to bring me back to the gym for yoga classes and light training. Going back to the gym only exacerbated my discomfort. Externally I seemed flexible but I held a lot of internal tension. It was time for me to follow the toe-to-head Fascianation

Method of self-massage routinely. I incorporated a breast rolling step for myself. Lo and behold! My breast tissue density went back to normal and I had no recurrence of polyps after surgical scraping for removal. At the time two of my friends who also had uterine polyps had their polyps surgically removed but months later more polyps grew and both friends required further treatment. The polyps were burned away, but ultimately each friend underwent a hysterectomy to rectify recurring uterine polyp issues. Rolling my lower abdomen assured me that healing oxygen and nutrients were getting to my tissues. My ovarian cyst reabsorbed. My allergies subsided. My neck stiffness went away after three days of whole-body rolling and my upper back pain and stiffness freed up after a few weeks. My shoulder pain was alleviated after a few days of rolling but took a couple of months to relieve permanently because I kept reversing my gains with my sleeping position, which I eventually learned to change. I felt that I hacked my body's immune system!

In 2012, Anthony and I felt that our hours of servicing people and projects that required repetitive and mundane tasks were not for naught! That year, a book comprised of studies and publications by a consortium of renowned clinicians, manual therapists, and scientists in several disciplines, was published. This book, *Fascia: The Tensional Network of the Human Body*, edited by experts in their fields, Robert Schleip, MA, Ph.D., Thomas Findley, MD, Ph.D., and Peter Huijing, Ph.D., was like Anthony's bible. Anthony finally had a one-stop resource. The reference book allowed Anthony to connect the client experience dots to profound truths about the tension and stress of the body. Around the same time, I started applying my years of lab expertise maintaining functional and healthy tissues systems to explain some of the things going on with Anthony's clients. I began to understand the healing success from rolling out clients toe to head regularly. The routine rolling program was like housekeeping. Rolling on the more rigid roller was like deep cleaning the body. Rolling regularly promoted fluid flushing and fluid balance. Re-establishing order and maintaining a neutral environment allows the body systems to work in concert with each other. The neutral environment restores the body's capacity to self-heal. You can imagine what our dinner conversations were about.

Our ideas were supported by real science! We weren't crazy! We weren't grasping at straws. That year, Anthony and I were fortunate to become founding members of The Fascia Research Society. Soon after, Anthony designed and developed The Fascianator in our backyard. We first tried using chair cushion foam, polyester batting, then yoga mats for the padding around a PVC pipe. We tried different adhesives like rubber cement, glues, and epoxies that didn't hold up in longevity tests. The adhesive property couldn't withstand the high temperatures of storage in the heat of a closed car in Hawaii.

Our first big sale of the early stage Fascianators was sold to a local chiropractor for retail sale. Soon after finalizing our final Fascianator design and product, the Tripler Army

Medical Center's Interdisciplinary Pain Management Center started teaching the self-care method. Since then, Waianae Coast Comprehensive Health Center and more medical institutions and academic institutions have begun teaching The Fascianation Method to their instructors and patients. Today our products are retailed in natural health stores, local gyms, and yoga studios in Hawaii. We also retail on Amazon.com. Fascianator Rolling classes are taught at Marriott Vacations Worldwide at Ko'Olina Resort as part of their clubTHRIVE program. ClubTHRIVE is an innovative program designed to help guests' physical and mental well-being and break the stress of daily life that many carry with them on vacation.

We hope for everyone to de-stress, thrive and explore our self-care innovation. We are training acupuncturists, massage therapists, yoga instructors, personal trainers, physical therapists, martial arts instructors, and caretakers The Fascianation Method. We have instructors in eleven states, Japan, and Sweden. We have been asked to participate in a proposed clinical research study funded by the Rheumatology Research Foundation. We are delighted that physicians, physical therapists, and chiropractors use The Fascianator and even refer their patients to see us.

Chapter 3:
Reset Your GPS

"When it is obvious that the goals cannot be reached, don't adjust the goals, adjust the action steps."
– Confucius

"If you can't fly then run, if you can't run then walk, if you can't walk then crawl, but whatever you do you have to keep moving forward."
– Martin Luther King Jr.

Are you ready to get in the driver's seat and behind the wheel to pain free living? You have the power to steer your health in the direction you want. Reset your GPS so that you avoid the detours that can delay your healing. The Fascianation Method is a methodical approach that changes you from the inside out organically and naturally. We work from within and work with the current state of your body.

We do not cut you open and surgically add or remove parts. We avoid pills and injections that mask the pain. We guide you to modify your beliefs and behavior which will enable you to remodel your internal environment. Behavior and belief are crucial factors that caused your chronic pain to begin and can prevent future pain from materializing to a chronic problem. If you use our methodical approach for pain relief, you will transform yourself from accepting your suffering to feeling exceptional!

Prioritize yourself. You have to make time for *you* and stop putting your needs on the back burner. Being busy is a way to numb yourself so that you won't have time to address your own needs, one of which is your need to resolve your chronic pain. Sometimes the numbing temporarily thwarts the worrying. It's common for people to be too occupied because they don't want to delve back into the world of dealing with their own issues or creating more challenges – more time off, more painful therapy, and more throwing spaghetti at the wall to see what sticks. Healing starts with awareness and, yes, self-love. For some, self-love is embraced. For others, it is difficult. Self-love is courageous because you have to face *everything* about yourself. You have to dig deep into the trenches. You have to start with fresh, nourishing soil and fix yourself from your roots on up.

You only have one body and that one body is the vessel through which you are helping others. We've all heard the idiom "take care of yourself before you take care of others." On an airplane flight, adults are told to put on their oxygen mask before their child's mask. If the adults don't have enough oxygen reaching their brain, how successful will they properly fit their child's oxygen mask? How will you continue to take care of others if you don't find a solid solution for your chronic pain? Is taking care of others an activity you'll have to eliminate if you don't fix your pain issue? Honor your worth and do not see self-care as a chore. I recognize that "me" time can sometimes feel like a chore and that needs to be re-framed. Focus on fixing your problem and don't get overwhelmed by the small stuff, those imaginary confrontations in your head. Feeling good is not a trivial thing. Feeling good is worth your precious time.

Make your mission not only to liberate your body from pain but also to learn_about your body. Rediscover your body. During massage therapy, you show up to your appointment and can check out and fall asleep while your body is being worked on. If you're able to stay awake, you'll realize that you had sensitivities in your body that you didn't know were tightness or tenderness. Many of my clients come on board only knowing *of* their body; not knowing *about* their body. When I cue them to bend down to try to touch their toes, most will bend down by curving the middle of their back (thoracic spine). When I cue them to keep their spine's normal curvature while bending down, they don't know where the normal curvatures should be and if they have normal or abnormal curvatures.

I encourage you to stand in front of a mirror with your arms at your sides. Observe your whole body from head to toe. Is one shoulder higher than the other? I'm guessing that the shoulder of your dominant arm is lower than that of the non-dominant arm. Are your collarbones level or is one collarbone higher than the other? Do they slant diagonally? Are your hips level? Now turn to the side and observe the curvature in your neck, upper back, and low back. Is your head aligned with your shoulders? An average head weighs around ten pounds. Forward head posture can be like having a fifteen-pound to forty-pound head. My neck and upper back hurt just thinking about that additional load that the neck and upper back can carry all day. Postural deviations undoubtedly play a part in chronic pain.

Form the habit to use The Fascianator and The Fascianation Method of the self-care just as regularly as you use a hairbrush. Some of our clients call fascial care an addiction! I've seen The Fascianator rolling habit form in as little as two weeks, but typically it takes two to three months to develop. Understand that everybody, meaning *every body*, has a different story. We have all endured different experiences and those damaging experiences causing physical and emotional stress and trauma are held in our tissues. If you have any reservations about following the methodology, do what you can. Do not let negative self-perceptions inhibit your motivation. Some clients feel incompetent or not physically fit enough when starting their program. If you are still reading this book, you have the competence. If you can sit on a couch or find a way to lie down safely and get back up safely, you are fit enough for the program. Allow yourself patience to develop the new skills in the program. The majority of beginners feel like a fish out of water.

JacquieMarie, a 72-year-old semi-retired dental hygienist of 52 years, attended our weekly class. JacquieMarie tried multiple healing modalities; physical and spiritual to manage her chronic pain. She modified all fifty-two positions of The Fascianation Method during her first month of classes. Her tenderness, joint instability, strength, and flexibility posed many challenges, but she had the determination to reap the benefits that she witnessed her friends reap. JacquieMarie showed up with her yoga mat and Fascianator, took the time to get comfortable working with the new tool, and listened to her body's feedback. After her third month of doing what she could, JacquieMarie increased her range of motion, had more mental clarity, and self-treated her headaches that she was told were caused by structural damage from twelve spinal injuries. JacquieMarie is more optimistic about getting older because she is using The Fascianation Method as her roadmap for her new self-care journey. Take some time to get comfortable. Make stable modifications that you feel are necessary. Work at your own pace. You can gradually add more steps of the program as your mind and body receive positive feedback. When you feel improvements in your body or quality of life, you will understand the value of whole body rolling and self-care and will be motivated to be more thorough.

Working with a coach will keep you accountable for actualizing your practice to achieve your goal. A coach can help you determine and eliminate disruptors of your progress. A coach will also help you realize your successes that you may not have been aware you've achieved. A coach will notice improved gait, posture, and new alignment. We have clients leaving class walking away without their canes. We have clients getting up from the ground twice as fast as they had initially stood up. If you don't have a coach, take the time to self-evaluate. Journaling works well for tracking progress and looking for patterns. Writing about your process will keep you engaged and more aware of the state of your body. Take inventory of how your mind and body feel before and during each practice and how your body responded to the practice. Did you notice disparities between one side of the body and the other? Did you cramp during your practice? Did your body crave more water? Do you have more endurance throughout the day? Did you have the biggest bowel movement the day after your first rolled your gut? Do you sleep better at night after you roll?

Seek social support to make forming the habit easier. Try to find a program buddy or create a meet-up group with like-minded people where you are seen and understood by others. You will know that you matter. It's motivating to see that other people are investing quality time in themselves. Fascianation Method classes have become many peoples' go-to events for connection and fellowship. It's uplifting to know that despite your differences, you share the similar goals of realignment, living chronic pain free, having more energy, and having joy for the rest of your prime and throughout your golden years.

Develop a positive mindset. Make today the first day of the rest of your life. While you're reading this book, you may be thinking, how the heck is this "rolling" and a new self-care program going to fix the things causing your intermittent and chronic pain? Perhaps a higher power has led you to find these alternative methods to relieve your pain. You have the ultimate control to react to what's presented to you and make the right decisions to improve yourself. Your mind may require mental metamorphosis. We have strategies that you can follow to break self-sabotaging behaviors and establish new brain patterns that foster positivity, a key mindset in achieving physical change. The placebo effect, gaining benefit from positive belief in treatment is real. The "nocebo effect" is also real. Having negative expectations of treatment can negatively impact progress and recovery. Focus on being productive, celebrate your successes, even small ones.

Continue to use this book as a resource. Continue the new connection with your body even after you achieve significantly more balanced physical, mental, and emotional states. Don't just address fascial care with rolling. I will discuss other modes of self-care that you should incorporate into your new health management lifestyle to maintain presence and awareness of your body. Your body is a biological system, always in flux and subject to ever-changing circumstances.

Chapter 4:

Free Your Mind

"Honor the Past, Release It,
Live the Present, Embrace It
Create the Future, Ignite It"
– Bonnie Lee Mahler

Since you're reading this book, you are probably unsatisfied with the care that you've received. You are seeking a solution to fix the cause of your suffering. You've sought out care, you've received orders to avoid the activity that results in pain, your imaging tests and nerve tests show no problems, you've been given pain pills or nerve blocks and completed weeks of physical therapy, but you still have daily pain. Surgery, exploratory or an -otomy (to cut into) or -ectomy (surgical removal) of some sort might have been recommended, but you're not ready for that. In this new world of innovation and incredible technological advances, it's shameful and an injustice to humanity to not be able to determine the root of chronic pain that millions of people endure. It seems to me that there are not enough round table discussions when it comes to patient care and what the patient actually faces once she leaves the doctor's office. Society has invested in putting people on Mars, fast-tracking to the moon, and flying at forty thousand feet in a carbon fiber tube all while streaming Netflix, but modern Western medicine has failed to identify the root cause of most chronic pain. You may be reluctant to go for a second opinion because you don't want to rack up more time off of work, more medical bills, more insurance statements to interpret, and you don't want another health professional to suggest that your pain is primarily in your head. You are not crazy even if you are taking the mental health medications prescribed for your complaints of pain. You are probably psychiatrically normal, but you're worn down chasing your tail while caught up in the old paradigm for chronic pain relief. You're worn down because massage therapists have grumbled that your tissue is like leather and too thick. You wear your massage therapists down yet you're still without positive results. Before you feel doomed, I've got good news that will make you bounce back. Our paradigm uses care tactics, not scare tactics.

We live in an unfair world. Although things didn't go the way you planned or wished with your therapy, you can still push yourself forward to have the pain free life that you deserve. If you focus your actions on growth and not just pain relief, you will make better things happen for you and not let things happen to you. Sometimes our dominant thoughts shaped by past experience get in the way of progress. We settle for status quo. Running on autopilot leaves us stuck and often unenergetic. Our thoughts and words are powerful. To maintain forward and resilient steps toward your goal, you may have to do a little brain housekeeping or mental conditioning.

Honor the past. Accept your experience. I don't think a time machine to change history is down Elon Musk's product pipeline, so stop sabotaging your future with negative thoughts from the past. You can't change time gone by. Release the negative feelings of your previous journey to resolve your chronic pain. By holding on to the beliefs that no longer serve you, you are mentally hoarding. Letting go of the negative emotions will create space for better opportunity. Negative emotions can weaken the immune system. I know that this is easier said than done. Our brain has a negativity bias. It's believed that holding on to negativities is a protective mechanism to keep us from dangers and harm's way. Negativity can spark worry and fear, and the combination of negativity and fear is a principal factor for overwhelm and misalignment. Even if you consciously eradicate negative thoughts, the subconscious mind can leave imprints of negative thought patterns in your deep tissues. Sometimes this is seen as poor posture but sometimes emotional holdings in the deep tissues are never apparent. The Fascianation Method can help tap into the deep tissue where emotional trauma is stored, buried, or repressed. I'll discuss this in later chapters.

Live in the present. Don't dwell on your limitations in areas you want to improve. Make every day you wake up an opportunity to work toward your dream come true. Do you have a morning ritual that recalibrates your mind, or do you unmindfully run on autopilot after you awaken and stumble out of bed? Upon waking, there are key things that I want you to add to your morning routine to set you up for the day's success. I prefer you do them right away; after you pee, before your morning caffeine buzz, and certainly before you pick up your phone or open your email! For most people, those distractions can wait ten minutes!

Meditate: Meditation is mind training that has been practiced for over five thousand years and has many forms and many purposes. Meditation can bring your brain to an idling state, allowing you to clear cerebral congestion including unwanted thoughts, and trains you to focus in the moment. It helps reduce stress and anxiety. Sit in a quiet space, sit upright in a chair or cross-legged if that's comfortable, close your eyes, and turn your attention away from the outside environment to your mind. Inhale slowly through your nose and exhale through your nose if you can, or mouth. Focus on your breathing; calm inhalation and calm exhalation. If your mind wanders in a parade of thoughts in your head, be aware but non-judgmental of those thoughts, emotions, and sensations of the present moment. Always bring your focus back your breathing and allow those thoughts to passively stream away. The aim is to be mindful but to not grab those thoughts and emotions and engage with them. If you are new at meditation, spend at least five to ten minutes practicing this relaxation and self-awareness technique before moving on to the next step. Meditation relaxes the mind and actually relaxes the fascia. Meditation can also be spiritual.

There are many resources available to help you fine-tune your meditation practice. Digital guided meditations are a great place to start. I recommend starting with the following free guided meditation by Dr. Bernie Siegel, which can be found on YouTube.

Overcome Life Stress and Strains with Dr. Bernie Siegel
https://youtu.be/l-7ttCJqGt8

This guided meditation is a little over twenty minutes long, which I think is the perfect duration of daily meditation that you should aspire to practice as a beginner.

Practice gratitude: Continuing from your meditation, think of one new thing that you are thankful for. Life isn't perfect, but recognize what you have. You have breath. You have eyesight. Make deposits into your feel-good bank and this will set you up for success to have more positive feelings. Reflect on it. Every day you wake up, you are blessed with another day to connect with another person. Who are you thankful for? Why are you grateful for that connection? Practicing gratitude can help you find more meaning, happiness, and motivation to strive.

Set an intention: Decide how you want to feel that day. Do you want to feel strong? Do you want to feel influential? Do you want to feel loved? Set your intention or determination of how you will feel throughout the day. Aim for your reactions, decisions, and actions to achieve that intention. Did you know that intention in medical terms is defined as a process or manner of healing?

Visualize success: Use the power of visualization to set yourself up for a good day. If you could snap your finger and no longer have chronic pain, what would you be doing? What is the scenery? What is the temperature? Who are you with? What are you wearing? You can also visualize positive outcomes for tasks and events that you will be faced with during your day. Visualize tension and darkness leaving your body while you roll your pain away. Many professional athletes imagine situations and plays before their performance or game. Brain activity during visualization is actually firing similarly to when the muscles are actually being used. Similar to physical practice, creating the familiarity reinforces brain patterns that create change. Imagery is very powerful.

Affirmations: Find positive affirmations and recite them. Positivity reinforces the nervous system and can initiate changes from inside out. Look in the mirror and say "I'm Number One! No one can do this for me but me!" You can even write affirmations on sticky notes and leave a note on your bathroom mirror, on the book you are reading, on your fridge, car dashboard, or work desk. Sometimes what's in our heads gets lost in the daily grind shuffle, so visual reminders are helpful. If you are not big on sentences of affirmations, start with displaying one word. Some examples are "joy", "freedom", or "tranquility". Just one positive word can have power in fostering hope and faith in your healing journey.

Take these daily steps to dispel old habits and programming. We can gracefully shake the hampering sensitivities that shape us from our past. Do you know someone who is constantly complaining, discussing the negativity in bad things that happen, and who forecasts tragic events that we have no control over? Do you notice that this person attracts problems and negativity? Keep your distance from this person! Don't get caught up in this person's ego game or your own ego game! Stay in control of your own energy. Condition the environment that you can control to give you more peace and more healthy power. Changing your outlook and how your mind operates is not an easy feat for most. It takes practice to improve. With practice comes experience and experience develops wisdom about your own mind, body, and soul. It may take one month or several months to incorporate the steps in your mindset ritual. It may also take unfamiliar, extraordinary effort and firm faith. It's scientifically proven that human beings have great plasticity—our minds, our tissues, even our genetic expression has incredible potential for change. Hang in there!

Chapter 5:

What's Fascia and Why Should I Care?

*"When we look at any one thing in the world,
we find it is hitched to everything else."*
– John Muir

*"The moment one gives close attention to anything,
even a blade of grass, it becomes a mysterious,
awesome, indescribably magnificent world in itself."*
– Henry Miller

I hope that you kind of like science. I hope you get my drift and don't drift from reading because fascia, though complex, is really fascinating and *extremely* vital to your physical and mental health!

If you've never thought of fascia as an organ, you're not alone. Fascia was recently classified as an organ system in 2012. There are many definitions of fascia and more than one school of thought on fascia, so I'll discuss some of the basics. It's both a type of connective tissue and an organ system that touches all of the other organs. Historically in the US, fascia has been a target tissue for treatment by osteopathic medicine doctors in the 1890s and bodyworkers as early as the 1940s.

Interestingly, even today, fascia is an emerging scientific field and rarely discussed as the culprit for chronic pain and dysfunction by allopathic healthcare professionals. Most modern Western Medicine practitioners do not assess fascia. In 2017, Anthony and I were invited to present our self-care method to over ninety physicians at Kaiser Permanente Hawaii's Professional Development Day. We asked what the audience knew about fascia. They had heard of apparent fascial structures that they learned about in anatomy when they were in medical school. For example, the plantar fascia at the bottom of the foot. They were aware that fascia surrounds muscles (also known as myofascia). Surprisingly the majority of the clinicians didn't know that fascial layers are the continuous network that surrounds our nerves, bones, blood vessels, and lymphatic vessels as well as penetrates, interconnects, and affects the health of *all* our organs. Fascia connects all of our seventy to eighty trillion cells. The expansive soft tissue scaffolding maintains the body's three-dimensional structure, regulation, and nourishment. It has an overarching role in homeostasis, the state of internal stability in living organisms. Perhaps because fascia is body-wide and not easily separated from other anatomical structures, its presence is not obvious; thus, its relevance to sickness was previously overlooked for hundreds of years in current Western medical science.

When I'm really congested and my nasal passages have been inflamed all day, I become lethargic. It should be evident that my body is taxed due to lack of oxygen in my tissues. But because oxygen is everywhere around me and I can't see, taste, smell, or feel oxygen gas, I forget about the concepts of oxygen fueling my body.

Depending on where the fascia is in the body, it will have different densities and appearances. If you've seen raw meat, you're familiar with deep fascia. It's that white fibrous sinew and slippery mucousy stuff that surrounds and penetrates the meat. If you pull the meat apart, the fascia resembles spider webbing. On a microscopic level, a cross section of the fascia of muscle or meat looks like a body-wide honeycomb of irregularly shaped silky pockets and tubes containing the individual muscle fibers.

If you're vegetarian, I have a very simplified example of fascia's continuity throughout its different layers. I want you to think about the structure of an orange. An orange has multiple layers and segments: rind, zest, pith, lith, and locule, which surrounds the juicy pulp. You can clearly see that all of these layers are actually one continuous structure.

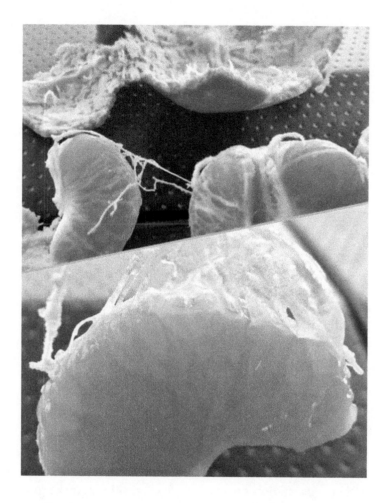

Fascia is an engineering marvel because it can withstand great tensional forces within the environment, like a skyscraper or suspension bridge. Healthy fascia is durable, elastic, and resilient. Fascia consists of three main components: fibers, cells, and a watery and gelatinous matrix in which the cells are suspended. This extracellular matrix is a cocktail of substances produced and secreted by fibroblasts, the cells of fascia. The extracellular matrix has essential functions which influence cell behavior. It helps regulate intracellular signaling and cell-to-cell cross talk. The matrix also protects cells from strong tensional forces, serves as the gate control for nutrients, and serves as a physical barrier to bacteria. Collagen and elastin, which hold lots of water are fascia's main fibrous components. Hyaluronic acid is the slippery part of the matrix that attracts and holds water. Do collagen and hyaluronic acid ring a bell? Google those biologic components and you'll see millions of beauty and nutrition ads that advertise collagen and hyaluronic acid for skin elasticity and anti-aging. Just as we consider healthy skin being firm, elastic, and moisturized skin, healthy fascial layers are strong, elastic, and hydrated. The elasticity and malleability of fascia enable fascia to withstand strong compression and stretch forces while returning to its original form and retaining its shape. The watery nature or viscosity of fascia allows the tissue to have a lubricant function.

Fascia is referred to as the body's tensional network and is now considered our most loaded sensory organ system. Other sensory rich organs are the eyes, skin, and the gut. Fascia contains millions of sensory receptors (structures that receive stimuli) including free nerve endings called mechanoreceptors. These receptors respond to mechanical tension like compression and stretch. This sensory and feedback mechanism by which cells convert mechanical stimulus to chemical or electrical messages is called mechanotransduction. It's so amazing that external force can exert its effect down to the cell's nucleus, where our DNA code is converted into instructions to make proteins and other functional molecules. Tension can actually modify our gene expression.

Fascia is involved in every movement we make and healthy fascia is a balance game; a literal balance game. Stiff, dry, and thickened fascia modulate vibrational messaging, biochemical messaging and cellular communication. It can affect proprioception, which is the sense of knowing where the body is in space, where your body is when you move. Fascial proprioceptors (specialized mechanoreceptors) respond to stretch and advise your brain of your positioning during movement. If fascia is too stiff, your perception can be off, affecting your limb position and joint movement. When stepping on a curb, you want your heel to first land on the curb, but if your tissues are inflexible you might instead stub your toes on the curbside. Your body doesn't properly respond to your brain's command. You fail to lift your toes high enough before you strike the curb. The amount of effort you think you need to properly position your body is off, so you miss the mark. You may even lose your balance.

Fascia holds about four gallons of water or interstitial fluid (water that bathes the outside of our cells and vessels) and behaves like a sponge. When we load our muscles, water is squeezed out of the fascia. When we release the load, more water rushes into the surroundings and penetrates fascia. This tissue hydration and flushing of waste product and toxin buildup trapped in our tissues are vital to maintain a non-stagnant, non-fermentative environment. After hand-washing the dishes, would you leave your sponge sopping wet with old dishwater until you do the next load of dishes or do would you wring out the old water in the sponge? To get a better feel of how fascia behaves, here's an exercise. Wet a new cellulose sponge, wring it out, and let it dry in the sun. Observe and feel the sponge after it has dried. It's stiff and shriveled. Now take the sponge, put it in bowl of water, watch it soak up the water and expand. Notice that the hydrated sponge goes back to its original shape and dimensions. You want your fascia to be like the damp sponge that retains its shape, dimensions, and receptor functionality. Hydrated tissue maintains the proper contact that it has with surrounding structures.

If you tend toward a sedentary lifestyle, there is less tissue flushing and more cellular waste product buildup in the environment. Poor circulation can cause edema and edema can cause a tensional shift in the fascia, which can then affect the inflammatory response in the environment. Also, with little movement, over time the fascial fibers will stiffen and lose their elasticity. Collagen fibers, which are oriented in particular angles, also become disorganized. An active youth will have myofascia that resembles a fishnet stocking. The individual collagen fibers are crimped and lined up parallel. The myofascia of a sedentary adult will look more like steel wool. The individual collagen fibers lack the crimp or spring-like structure and are not lined up parallel. Imagine gliding your fingers through untangled hair versus a tangled balled-up mess. Lack of movement overtime reduces overall mobility and can lead to injury like a strain, sprain, or tear. On the flip side, too much activity without proper tensional release like routine stretching or frequent bodywork/massage can also lead to stiff fascia, soft tissue adhesions, fascial layer cross-links (think molecular glue which prevents fibers gliding and receptor accessibility) and muscle fiber knots also known as trigger points, all which lack resilience. Think about knots in wood. Knots are formed on tree trunks after branches fall off of a live tree and the tree continues to grow. The knot is similar to scar tissue. If you try to drive a nail into the knot, you'll see that it's not an easy task at all. The resistance even bends nails. Driving a nail into a healthy part of the wood is easier.

Stiff or taut musculature around the joints decrease the space within the joint capsule. This contributes to cartilage wear and tear and compression of the joints. Cartilage is made of specialized cells that produce pliable matrix proteins. If joint compression is sustained the shock absorbing connective tissue and joint lubricating synovial fluid around the joint dry out. Over time this chronic compression leads to degeneration. You want the fascia surrounding your joint capsules to retain hydration and viscosity to avoid cartilage on bone or bone on bone friction.

Fascia transmits and absorbs forces like springs and shock absorbers. Healthy fascia evenly distributes forces and loads over the whole muscle. Myofascial restrictions can exert around 2,000 pounds per square inch of tensile pressure on pain sensitive structures. Can you imagine feeling the compression of 2,000 pounds on any square inch of your body? That's the equivalent of being over 4,613 feet under water. Those values reflect the chronic pain that clients describe as glass shards poking their thighs or even their face. On a pain scale of one to ten, how would you rate that pain level? If the pain is chronic, I describe the pain level as off the chart.

Let's discuss the compression of an important type of structure in our body. The structure is a neurovascular bundle, a package of nerves, arteries or veins, and lymphatic vessels that travel together throughout the body. Neuro=nerve. Vascular=vessels (artery, vein, and lymphatic). Bundle= together. Imagine electricity wires traveling through a house. The wires have to penetrate walls to get to the various rooms. These neurovascular bundles penetrate various sheets of the superficial and deeper fascia in around your body to get from the trunk to the arms and legs.

Hydrated and Pliable

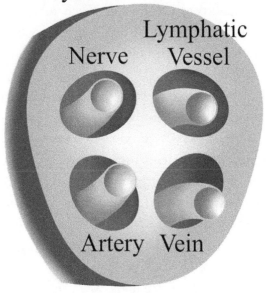

Stiff

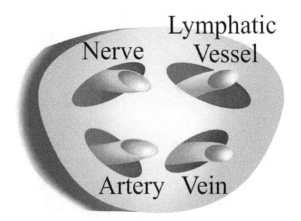

In the images on the previous page, each schematic represents a neurovascular bundle. Each tube represents a conduit: An artery, which delivers oxygen and nutrient-rich blood throughout the body; a vein, which returns de-oxygenated blood to the heart; a lymphatic vessel, which works closely with blood vessels and transports lymph fluid (containing white blood cells, excess or bad proteins, possibly bacteria) away from the tissues toward the heart; and a nerve that carries sensory information. Refer to the schematic of the neurovascular bundle surrounded by hydrated and pliable fascia. Notice the space and compression around the vessels. Refer to the schematic of the neurovascular bundle surrounded by stiff, dry fascia. There is less space around the vessels, and with 60,000 miles of blood vessels in the body, we believe that the dry fascia can compress a lot of the vessels. The compression squeezes the blood vessels that deliver oxygen-rich or deoxygenated blood and leads to poor blood circulation. The squeezing of the nerve can cause neuropathy, numbness, tingling, weakness, or idiopathic pain, which is chronic pain of unknown origin. Squeezing the lymphatic vessel inhibits fluid filtration and fluid balance; it can cause edema, swelling, and even blood pressure issues. On the pain scale, how would you rate numbness due to a compressed nerve or blood vessel? For most people, that would be hard to evaluate and describe.

A nagging injury that you can't seem to shake is likely due to fascia stiffening to protect the injured area. During injury and even just assault (banging your leg against a doorframe), there's an interplay between the fascia and the immune response. Connective tissue is practically part of the immune system. Fascia's response to injury is a communication cascade, like an emergency phone call tree. This cascade causes swelling to splint/immobilize the joint as well as inflammation, which is white blood cells moving to the injury site. The white blood cells secrete chemicals. The swelling, chemicals, and inflammation compress nerves, causing pain. Some of the substances secreted cause fibroblasts normally around the site to transform into myofibroblast cells. Let's call these myofibroblast cells repairmen. The repairmen work to repair tissue at and around the injury site. As long as there's sustained aggravation or strain on the area, the repairmen try to heal by laying down collagen. If you don't rest the injury or if you move the injured area too much too soon, you cause assault to the damage. The repairmen keep working and keep laying down more collagen. This over-healing or dysregulated wound healing leads to scarring or fibrosis. If the balance is restored, the repairmen are instructed to breakdown scarring by breaking down collagen with an enzyme called collagenase.

With internal injuries, early fibrosis is usually not apparent with routine medical imaging tests. Conventional MRI lacks the sensitivity to detect the slow changes in the collagen structure and matrix proteins. You might immobilize the injured area for an extended period of time, which can also lead to stiff, disorganized fascia that can cause more problems down the road. We caution our clients about wearing an orthopedic boot for too long. Nagging injuries typically lead to fibrosis, compensatory movements, and postural deviations. As a personal trainer and movement specialist, I look for postural deviations and imbalance of bony landmarks like clavicles, shoulder blades, and ribs. The deviations lead to muscular imbalances, unstable joints, and inefficiency in movement and in fluid flow. When the fascia is moving smoothly, you are more aware, feel lighter, have better balance, less stagnation, and positive flow.

Have you ever heard of Rolfing Structural Integration? It's a form of manual therapeutic bodywork that was created by biochemist Dr. Ida Rolf. Ida Rolf was about 80 years ahead of her time because her therapy for poor posture targeted the fascial system. Ida called fascia the organ of posture. She stated that "fascial web connects and communicates throughout the body; thickened areas transmit strain in many directions and make their influence felt at distant points, much like a snag in a sweater. This is a mechanism through which reflex pressure points become manifest." Ida Rolf's beliefs explain why local soft tissue strains can alter skeletal alignment and movement. She knew that structural misalignments cause excess soft tissue tension, joint issues, and pain. Rolfing therapy involves multiple sessions of direct pressure and slow strokes to relieve fascial thickening. Rolfing doesn't get the popularity that it deserves because it is quite painful for most people.

The majority of our female clients around age fifty have shoulder joint annoyances that often progress to frozen shoulder. The mid-late forties is a great time to be wary of the intense one hundred pushups, one hundred burpees, or heavy dumbbell overhead press workouts. Even bowling turned out to be a health hazard for one of our clients. Be informed and be loving to your body! You want to condition and hydrate the fascia that surrounds your joints and neurovascular bundles. Incorporating a fascial care routine can help mitigate joint degeneration. Estrogen levels substantially decrease during peri-menopause and disappear after menopause. Decreased estrogen leaves us dry. The dryness permeates down to the fascial web's ground matrix. Current fascia research data suggests that hyaluronic acid levels decline with age and that the less estrogen women have, the greater chance the immune response to injury progresses to scar tissue formation or fibrosis. Research also shows that fibrosis starts in the neurovascular bundles, the bundles of our vessels, nerves, and lymphatics. That fibrosis might explain all the unexplained, often ignored or undetected health changes women feel in their mid-forties and beyond. In a nutshell, suboptimal healing is an effect of peri-menopausal and menopausal estrogen levels. A healthy self-care regimen should include routine fascial care!

Reconnecting with your fascia can affect your motivation, sense of well-being, and embodiment. Since the nervous system and the fascial systems are interwoven, relaxing the fascia can relax the nervous system. Studies show that relaxing the fascia around the abdominal area or pelvis can produce parasympathetic reflexes which are relaxing and help you chill out. A common saying to remember the parasympathetic system is that it helps you "rest and digest; feed and breed". Fascia contains interoceptors for sensing your internal physical and physiological state. Interoceptors help you determine if you're thirsty, hungry, hot, aroused, etc. If you unbind and unwind your fascia, you allow the massive amount of interoceptors to be exposed and available to receive and properly process biochemical messages. You will have a better sense of what's going on in your body. You'll have a better awareness of when you're hungry or when you have heartburn. Motion affects emotion: proprioception interplays with interoception. If you move, you can better control your emotion. Don't you feel happy when you're dancing or when you watch a dance performance? As kids, when we jumped up, down, and all around or hung upside-down on monkey bars, we were moving our organs around. Visceral fascia lines our organs. We are better situated when our visceral fascia gets some TLC – more oxygen and nutrient absorption and stimulating areas that become stiff and dry.

You now know fascia as an intricate physical fabric that can transfer information from one place to another. Fascia gets even more exciting because collagen has electrical properties and when collagen and other matrix substances interact with other molecules and cells in its environment, fascia becomes a body-wide electrical circuit. At rest, the average human gives off energy that can light a 100-watt lightbulb. This network of circuity is a dynamic energy system and the target system for many holistic energy medicine healers. In Chinese medicine, healing takes place along the energetic channels that are called meridians. The meridians functionally connect all parts of the body. The meridians are where the invisible Qi or bioelectric energy flows. Sickness and disease can result from blockages or stagnation of the Qi. Tom Meyers, an authority in the fascia world, developed the idea of myofascial meridians, which have much overlap with Chinese acupuncture meridians. In acupuncture, the skin puncturing needle targets the collagen in connective tissue points. Fibroblasts become stimulated and the cascade of healing events commence. Tissue stiffness and fascial restrictions cause congestion and energy blocks. Like stiff fascia, rigid belief systems can make you inflexible and stuck in thought patterns that do not foster positive energy flow and shifts within our physical being. The energy of unresolved emotional issues and trauma often store in the deep fascia. The emotional holding can cause stagnation, acidity, and chronic contracture and inflammation where people tend to carry their stress. Vibrational therapies such as light, sound, and heat therapy coupled with good bodywork can heal tissue distortions and unclog energy blocks.

Does it now make sense why you should care about fascia? Fascia can have incredible energy storage and amazing self-healing properties. If you take care of your fascia, your fascia will take care of you! If you enable your fascia to flow, you will even feel a new degree of embodiment and uncover your natural healing ability. Addressing fascial restrictions has healed our clients' common aches and pains associated with aging, sedentary lifestyle, repetitive stress injury, and wear and tear. Their ability to gain freedom from chronic pain and mobility restrictions have lifted their spirits. Because fascia is everywhere, it's an excellent medium for whole body health care.

Margaret, a Biodynamic Craniosacral Therapist and Embodiment Coach, was delighted to share her early experience with her Fascianation Method journey. Margaret had been taking care of her fascia with sporadic massage and daily Chi Gong shaking, but she didn't feel that those modalities were enough to achieve fascial equilibrium. She kept feeling increasing constriction in her upper torso and arms.

As she rolled, she felt a wonderful sense of warmth in her body that she attributed to improved blood and lymphatic circulation. That great warmth brought much presence and awareness into her body.

Once in a while, she encountered more tender body areas; places of stagnation, or congestion. She knew that she needed to allow the local pinches and congestions to soften because release in one area of the body can feel like a full system release.

A few minutes into the practice, she felt her autonomic nervous system begin to rebalance. She felt her vagus nerve kick in, which provided a wonderful sense of warmth spreading to her chest and belly. In Margaret's words:

"That's the body's way of saying all is well; you can rest, digest, and heal now. The adrenals can catch a break and a wonderful silence and clarity enter the mind. This can potentially trigger powerful intrinsic rebalancing processes. Few times after the exercise I noticed micro-movements in my body. This was my body allowing me to release past trauma. It is important to stay with the micro-movements and allow them to come to completion on their own. It may be accompanied by emotional sensations and just letting it all wash through you is a tremendous gift from yourself to you. So, I can say that this system of self-care supports trauma release processes leading to more balanced physical, emotional, and mental state."

After Margaret's first Fascianation Method rolling class her joint mobility increased by at least twenty percent. After three weeks of rolling (full body every three days) her posture and flexibility greatly improved, she maintained upper back tensional relief as shown by her shoulder position in resting state. Her shoulders were at least one inch lower than before using The Fascianation Method.

Not all self-myofascial release rollers are the same! If you do not already have The Fascianator roller, you can order one at www.thefascianator.com. Mention our book and we'll hook you up!

Chapter 6:

The Fascianation Method of Self-Care

"Don't be trapped by dogma - which is living with the results of other people's thinking. Don't let the noise of others' opinions drown out your own inner voice. And most important, have the courage to follow your heart and intuition."
– Steve Jobs

The Fascianator roller is used for The Fascianation Method of self-care. The Fascianator roller was mindfully designed to fit in anatomical spaces so that your spine stays aligned when rolling. The rigidity of the roller can be intimidating at first, especially if you have never used a roller, or even if you have used a foam roller but still have very tight tissue. Some people's knots and adhesions are harder than the foam roller. Using a foam roller in such case is like using a dull knife to cut through tomato skin. To elicit the body's response of tensional release in very tight tissues, the rigidity of The Fascianator is necessary. To achieve the wringing effect of the waste water in your tissues and to move the waste fluid to the organs for filtration, you need the pressure coupled with the slow rolling motion. Remember that mechanical pressure is necessary to start the intracellular and intercellular communication cascade.

General Rules for Rolling with The Fascianator Roller

1. Perform whole body rolling at least two times per week.
2. Do slow, controlled deep breathing (in through your nose if possible and out through your mouth) while you roll.
3. Do not spend more than three minutes maximum rolling the same area.
4. All techniques are to be performed on both sides of the body to neutralize the tensional imbalances.
5. Drink plenty of water during and after you roll. You will need to flush out the toxins and waste products that were in your tissues.
6. Be cautious to roll after a recent injury. Wait seventy-two hours to roll after a painful injury.
7. Do not roll over areas of acute inflammation – areas that are swollen and red.

8. Do not roll over bursitis (fluid sacs between joints that are inflamed).

9. Do not roll over your ribs. Take special care to know where your two pairs of floating ribs (ribs not attached to your breast plate) are.

10. Do not roll over bony landmarks.

11. Do not roll where there are screws, rods, or a pacemaker.

12. Consult your physician before you start any new exercise program and if you have questions.

Part 1: Lower Body Rolling

By rolling the fascia in your lower legs you can improve your balance and eliminate issues caused by ankle or foot overuse. Common issues are tight ankles, cramping feet and toes, plantar fasciitis, heel pain, arch pain, bunions, crooked feet, hammer toes, tarsal tunnel syndrome, and bone spurs.

Rolling your lower legs will require some core, arm, and shoulder strength and stability. Don't worry if you can't get into the exact rolling positions right away. I offer "baby step tips" to follow until you have the ability to practice the progression. If the baby step tip is still too hard to follow, modify the baby step and adjust the time suggested to roll. Gently explore your ability and challenge yourself after you find the comfortable sweet spot.

Feet

You'll start by rolling your feet to unblock energy flow and increase circulation in your feet. There are thousands of nerve endings in the feet. If you roll the bottom of your feet, you stimulate communication through those nerves, which travel to different areas and organs of our bodies. Listen and feel for crackly sensations. You will break up crystalline deposits of uric acid, calcium, or inflammatory molecules in your feet. You will hydrate and untangle dry and bundled fascial fibers. The increased blood flow and circulation will help flush waste and toxin buildup out of your body.

Rolling Technique

You will roll one foot at a time. You can hold onto a chair for balance. Stay balanced by slightly bending the leg of your balancing knee. Start with your right foot on the Fascianator. Tilt your right foot in slightly toward your inner arch while pushing your arch into the roller for pressure. Slowly roll up to the ball of your foot and down to the bottom of your inner arch. Spend twenty seconds rolling this medial plantar fascia.

Shift your foot laterally to roll the lateral/outer arch. This is a whole different structure. For twenty seconds, slowly roll up and down the lateral arch. Apply different pressures and take note if it is more tender, more crackly, or more gritty than the inner arch. Next, shift your weight to the middle of your foot as your foot is laid flat on the roller. Roll down to the base of the foot to your heel. Spend twenty seconds rolling here. Switch to rolling the left foot.

Ponder

If you have plantar fasciitis you might be able to feel grittiness at the attachment of this tissue on the heel bone. Does it feel more tender or less tender rolling the left foot than the right foot? According to dominance, the non-dominant side has more tension than the weaker side. If you're very in tune with your body, you may notice that after rolling your right foot, your right foot has an easier time stabilizing while balancing to roll the left foot.

Some people wear expensive custom orthotics for their foot pain. Is what you put in your shoe going to fix the issues in your tissues or is the constant use of orthotics a crutch that prolongs the soft tissue problems?

There are about thirty joints in the foot. Imagine someone inside of your foot with a can of WD-40, spraying around every articulation. What is the net result? Your foot will feel looser. You will feel more balanced. By rolling both feet, you are finding where the tensional imbalances are and neutralizing those imbalances for improved function.

Calves

Posterior muscles of the lower leg between the knee and the ankles; above the Achilles tendon.

Rolling Technique

While in a seated position, put the thickest part of your right calf on The Fascianator. Face your toes up toward the ceiling. Stack your left leg on top of your right calf to add more pressure to the area you're rolling. While your hands are planted on the ground beside your hips, with proper posture, chest up, shoulders back and lift up your hips. Roll down to your Achilles tendon. Roll back up your calf to right below the knee. Try to relax your right foot while rolling. Spend twenty seconds rolling up and down the calf. If your wrists or shoulders feel strained, you do not have to lift your hips and rolling does not have to be continuous. Take breaks.

Wherever there are very tender points, keep the pressure on the tender spot for twenty seconds to force the knot to relax.

Repeat the rolling steps above, but turn your foot in to massage the inner head of your calves. Spend twenty seconds rolling the inner calf muscle then turn your foot out to roll the outer head of your calf. Remember to try and relax your feet!

Baby Step Tip

Instead of rolling up and down your legs with your hips up, place your calf on The Fascianator. Apply pressure (by pressing leg into The Fascianator or stack your legs for more pressure), swivel your leg left to right, horizontally massaging across the calf muscle fibers.

Repeat by repositioning different areas of your calf onto The Fascianator. Spend about twenty seconds rolling.

Posture Tips

Avoid putting all your weight on your shoulder joints by lengthening your spine and centering and straightening your ribcage. Chest up, shoulders back!

Ponder

Do not be alarmed if your foot starts trembling. Keep the pressure on your calf until the trembling subsides. Like driving, keep the pressure on the gas or the brake to maintain smooth driving. The stored tension in your calves is fighting a stretch reflex. Extended pressure elicits another physiological response called autogenic inhibition. When receptors perceive a certain level of tension in your muscle's tendon, your brain tells your muscle fibers to stretch or relax.

Tensional release in your calves can relieve problems felt in your feet! Calves have lots of sensory receptors (structures that receive stimuli) in them because we subconsciously rely on our lower legs to know our joint position to execute our movement.

When your calves are tight, you may feel chronic heel pain or effects of plantar fasciitis, inflammation of the tissue on the bottom of your foot. Loosening up your calves can also decrease lower back pain. Tight calves pull on the back of your upper leg, which pulls on your lower back. For those of you who wear high heels, does your lower back hurt after hours of standing in them? The static position is sustained muscle contraction. Imagine the contraction, the shortening of the calf fascia pulling on the hamstring, which is a force that pulls on the lower back fascia.

Veins and lymphatic vessels have one-way valves to prevent backflow. If veins are compressed, the one-way valves lose their integrity which results in varicose veins-- veins that are enlarged and have reflux blood flow.

After rolling both feet and calves, walk around and notice how your feet and gait feel. You may feel "lighter," as if you are walking with moon boots on. You may feel more grounded as your feet have better contact with the ground.

Fibularis

Muscle group below and to the side of the knee. Fibularis muscles allow lateral leg and foot movement and help to maintain balance while shuffling laterally. They are responsible for lateral mobility and stability of the ankle. Each leg has two fibularis muscles that start below the knee and go down the side of the leg. The muscles continue to become your tendons and continue to the bony protrusion on the side of your foot. From there, the connective tissue continues to wrap around the bottom of your heel and attaches to your toes.

Rolling Technique

Rolling your fibularis will be very tender. In a right-side plank position (right hip and right elbow on the floor, opposite hip facing the ceiling, using your left hand to help hold your body up) place your fibularis tissue right below your knee onto The Fascianator. To add more pressure, lift your hips off the ground. Avoid putting all your weight on your shoulder by lengthening your spine, and center and straighten your ribcage. In other words, do not collapse your chest. Slowly roll up and down about three to four inches for twenty seconds.

Baby Step Tips

Place your fibularis on The Fascianator, stack your legs, keep your hips on the mat, and slightly tilt your opposite hip down toward the floor and rotate your hip back to starting position toward the ceiling. You will do more rocking and tilting than rolling. Repeat for twenty seconds. You are massaging across your fibularis.

Ponder

Fibularis and Achilles tendon tightness can lead to pain where they connect to the bottom of the foot. Have you ever lost your footing and rolled your foot laterally, thus spraining your ankle? If your fibularis muscles are hydrated and pliable, you will be able to quickly roll your foot back to a normal walking position to absorb inconsistencies in uneven ground that you are walking on or avoid the tensional pull that can tear an ankle ligament.

Your toes may tingle while rolling your fibularis. The temporary tingling is nerve conduction because the nerve is deep under the muscle compartment. Your nerve may be waking up. Anthony and I each had clients who developed paraplegia after unfortunate accidents. After over five years and eight years of having no feeling in their feet and having been told that they will never feel their feet, sensation returned to their feet after a couple of months of regular Fascianator rolling.

Too much tension and inflammation can cause bone to grow. The bony prominence of the outside of the lower leg near the knee can grow. We see this often, even with youth that engage in multi-sport activities causing leg overuse.

Front of Lower Leg (Anterior Tibialis)
The tibialis anterior is attached to your shin bone, or tibia, and the base of your foot. It helps with lifting your toes back toward your foot.

Litmus test
Before rolling, place both calves onto the Fascianator. Rotate your feet at the ankle in a clockwise and counter-clockwise position. Note any stiffness and crackling of the ankles. After rolling your fibularis and anterior tibialis of both legs, rotate your ankles again and compare the stiffness before rolling and after rolling. After rolling, your ankle joints should have more space and the joint should feel looser when rotating your feet in circles.

Rolling Technique

Rolling your shins will be very tender. You will roll the shin opposite the side where you would feel shin splints. Starting in a crawling position on all fours, extend your right leg out, and place the outer front of your lower leg (anterior tibialis) on the roller. Slowly roll up and down about four inches for a total of twenty seconds. For more pressure, drop down on your elbows and stack your left leg over your right leg while you are rolling.

Baby Step Tips

Hold the Fascianator in your hands and use the Fascianator like a rolling pin to roll the outer front of your lower leg.

Ponder

Your toes may tingle while rolling your shins. The tingling is not a bad thing. It is better blood flow or communication in nerves strangled by tight fascia. When you feel uncomfortable sensations that are not sharp pains while rolling, reframe that "OW!" to "OH! I've found some areas of my body where I should spend quality time!

If you are a runner, avid walker, or sand or stair walker, you may have had shin splints – sharp stabbing pains or achiness in your shins. Remember that fascia can transmit two thousand pounds per square inch on pain-sensitive structures. Tight fascia of the shins can tug on the fascia lining the shin bone. We believe that tugging can cause bone spurs or can pull on the toes and cause toes to curl up. Modern treatment for curled toes is cutting the tendons of the toe to straighten the toe. Imagine the nerve damage or scar tissue that can follow. In our self-preservation process we roll, we don't cut!

In each lower leg, there is a neurovascular bundle that perforates through a fascial sheath that makes different compartments in the leg. Tight fascia can create dangerous pressure that compresses or pinches your neurovascular bundles. The excess pressure will result in poor circulation, impaired nerve conduction, swelling, and even poisoning of the tissue in the compartment.

Have you ever seen anyone whose lower leg bows out like bananas? Legs bowing out below the knee are called "banana calves". Tight lower leg muscles actually tug on the bones to cause the bone deformation.

Hamstrings
Your hamstrings include three muscles at the back of your thigh. They stabilize your knees.

Rolling Technique
Plant one foot on the ground. Place the back of the opposite thigh on the Fascianator, just above the knee. Do no lock your knee of the leg that you are rolling. Roll the outer hamstring up and down by turning the thigh outward. Roll from above the knee all the way up to under the gluteus maximus/butt. Roll the inner hamstring by turning the thigh inward. Proceed to roll up and down

from just above the knee all the way to under the butt. Switch to the other leg.

Baby Step Tips

Instead of lifting the hips off the ground, place the roller under the hamstring and rotate your thigh left and right. You will do more rocking than rolling. Push your hip and leg into the roller like you want to have a deep conversation with your fascia. Don't be afraid. If you've ever tried a foam roller, were you able to have as deep a conversation?

Ponder

Your hamstrings won't be as sensitive as your calves, so don't look for pain before you move on. Look for inconsistencies in your tissues. You want to feel where the issues of stickiness are. They are usually in between the two segments of the hamstring that are stacked one on top of the other. You want to spend time with the deepest muscle next to the femur. Your leg might involuntarily shake as the muscle is trying to resist the relaxation process. This is feedback that your tissue needs more attention. Don't wait until you feel leg or low back pain to address tight hamstrings. Tight hamstrings can cause low back pain and knee pain. I have seen several people rip their hamstrings off of their bone because they engaged in a very dynamic motion without properly conditioning their soft tissues. To avoid injury, soft tissues should have the elasticity to withstand certain force overload or dynamics.

Gluteals and Deep Hip Rotators

The target area to roll your gluteals is closer to your waist, not the apple bottom part of your butt cheeks. Rolling out your deep hip rotators, which span across your butt, will relax muscles that, if very tight or inflamed, could pinch your sciatic nerve.

Rolling Technique

Brace yourself and take deep breaths while rolling your hips rotators. These areas will scream at you your first few times rolling them! Try to relax into the position. Through practice, you will release the tension that your butt and hips store and your scream will become a purr.

Place your right elbow on the ground. Place your right hip on The Fascianator. Cross your right leg over your left leg (if you have a total hip replacement you should not cross your leg. Plant both feet on the floor, slightly bend your knees). For better support, make sure your left knee is bent and planted on the floor. Hold your right ankle and keep your chest up to ensure a stable shoulder. Roll up all the way to the upper hip. Do not roll too low, as it may cause you to fall off The Fascianator. Switch sides.

Baby Steps Tips

Carefully sit on the Fascianator. Keep your knees bent and feet planted on the floor. Let your legs to fall to the right side. Place your right elbow on the ground. Keep your chest up to stabilize the shoulder. Pushing with your feet, slowly roll all the way up to the upper hip and roll back to your start position. Do not roll too low, as it may cause you to fall off The Fascianator.

Posture Tips

Support your shoulder by keeping your chest up. Center and straighten your ribs.

Ponder

Tight gluteals and hips can contribute to low back pain as well as sciatica. Should you be getting back surgery right away if you have sciatic pain? Underneath your gluteals are 6 hip rotator muscles. The sciatic nerve runs between two of those muscles. Inflammation of two hip rotator muscles can compress the sciatic nerve and is a usual culprit for sciatica. Address your soft tissue around the problem area before resorting to surgery.

Inner Thighs/Adductors

In each inner thigh, there are five muscles attached from the hip to your knee.

Rolling Technique

Place the Fascianator in a longitudinal position. Start with your elbows on the mat and hips facing the mat. Place your inner thigh on the roller as close to a ninety-degree angle as possible and tilt your ankle up slightly. Be sure not to lay your body on the ground as you need your bodyweight to put enough pressure on the inner thighs. Lift your weight on the opposite toe so that you can push yourself into the roller. Press your inner thigh into The Fascianator and roll all the way up to the inner hip space. Turn in toward the pubic bone. That area will be sensitive. Switch sides.

Baby Step Tip

Sit on your mat and spread your legs out, making a V. You can also roll your inner thighs seated in a chair. Use the roller like a rolling pin to massage up and down your inner thighs. Do you feel more tender sensation closer to the knee joint or closer to the hip/groin? You probably never guessed that you had much tension stored in your inner thighs.

Ponder

Which inner thigh is telling you more of their secrets? Don't be surprised if you have knee issues and your inner thigh is very tender closer to your knee. Don't be surprised if you have sensitivity more towards the upper inner thigh where your femoral artery enters your thigh. You want to keep the fascia around your femoral artery pliable.

You have lymph nodes under the adductors. People with chronic inflammation have clogged nodes and lymphatic vessels. How do you think they are purging the toxins and metabolic waste if they don't roll or have frequent lymphedema massages or myofascial release treatments?

Quadriceps/Hip Flexors

You have four quadriceps muscles. These muscles attach to the knees and the hips.

Litmus Test

Perform the test before rolling and before switching to the other leg. Compare the rolled vs the unrolled leg. Lift your knee toward your chest. Safely try to lift as high as you can. After rolling, you'll see you can raise your knee higher than you think! Try the knee lift a couple of times, because your range of hip flexion should increase after rolling.

Rolling Technique

Roll one leg at a time. Place the roller on the front of your thigh near your knee. Proceed to roll your thigh towards your groin. Roll right before the crest of your pelvis area. Be sure to avoid any bony landmarks. Roll back down toward your knee. When you find a very tender spot, pause for about twenty seconds. This pause is vital to force tissue relaxation. Roll the inner quadricep muscle by pointing your toes out. You should feel your weight shift to the innermost quadricep muscle. Roll up towards your pelvis then back down close to your knee. Do a few passes. After you roll the middle of your thigh, tilt out about fifteen degrees to increase your pressure on your outer quadricep just next to your iliotibial (IT) band. Roll the outer quadricep all the way up to the side of your hip bone, and down to right above your knee, avoiding your bony landmarks. Switch sides. Men should take care to not roll over their privates!

Baby Step Tip

You can roll your quadriceps while seated in a chair. Use the Fascianator like a rolling pin. If you are able to roll on the ground, face your hips down and place both thighs on the roller. The tops of your feet should be face-down on the mat. Roll both legs at a time. After a few passes of rolling in this position, rotate your toes out and roll up and down your thighs. Pay close attention when rolling close to your knees. You may feel tender areas closer to your knee joint.

Ponder

Tight quadriceps will pull on the knee and can cause knee pain. Tight quadriceps will rub on the bony protrusion of the femur. Knee pain is felt in different areas relative to the patella, so take care to spend time rolling all four of your quadriceps muscles.

Tight hip flexors lead to an anterior pelvic tilt, which creates more spinal curvature, puts pressure on discs in between the lumbar vertebrae, and pulls on the nerve roots of your spinal cord. Remember that if your back hurts, your back may not actually be hurt. The tissue surrounding the area of pain might be stiff and dry. If you remove the imbalances of the spine, you will alleviate lower back pain and the pressure on the disc will decrease. The disc may come back in.

Abdominal Region

The abdominal area has a lot of complicated processes happening there. You have lots of organs in this area, like your intestines, diaphragm, reproductive organs, and of course miles of nerves and blood vessels which will really appreciate some tissue relaxation, TLC, and fresh oxygen.

Litmus Test

Exhale. Now take a slow deep breath in through your nose and notice where your breath stops. Take note of where you feel your breath stopped. After you roll your intestinal space, take another good deep breath in through your nose. Does it feel that you can breathe in deeper?

Rolling Technique

Point your finger to your belly button and bring the fingers across the sides of your torso until you feel your twelfth ribs, also known as the floating ribs. Make sure you *do not roll over these ribs*. To ensure you stay away from your ribs, *do not roll higher than your belly button!*

Lay prone, hips facing down, and position the right edge of the Fascianator on the *right* side/oblique area, *staying below* the belly button. Lean right, allowing the roller to sink into your tissue. Take a deep breath in and exhale, letting the abdominal muscles relax. Bend your left knee so that it's parallel to the roller. Crawl forward two to three inches until the Fascianator reaches the bladder. Crawl back down a few inches, avoiding your ribs. After a few passes, switch to the left side.

Move the edge of the Fascianator over to the left oblique and repeat the procedure on the left side. Bend your right leg for stability.

Ponder

Loosening up stiff tissues around the diaphragm in the abdominal area will help increase your lung capacity. Stiff abdominal tissue can lead to shallow breathing. If your transversus abdominus (your torso girdle) and diaphragm are too stiff and tight, your diaphragm can't lower and flatten to allow lung expansion.

Loosening up the stiff tissue around the bladder has helped our clients get more hours of uninterrupted sleep overnight because they no longer have to get up three to five times a night to relieve their bladders.

Ladies, rolling your lower abdomen can help regulate the balance of your reproductive organs. If you have cysts, polyps, fibroids, or severe menstrual cramps, roll your lower abdomen. Roll down to your pubis if that is not too painful. Restore balance caused by tension and inflammation around your female organs. Several of our female clients of fertile age yet unable to conceive were able to conceive after regularly rolling for a few months. Many clients have reported less vaginal dryness and finally unpainful intercourse. Several clients no longer have debilitating pain from ovarian cysts, especially bleeding ovarian cysts.

Gut health affects your whole body's health. You've rolled your intestinal area, so don't be surprised if you have a big bowel movement tomorrow. Mechanically move out the waste and toxins that can fester in your body, impede nutrient absorption, and create imbalances of the microbial flora in your gut. Your gut has good microbes that are essential and it also has invading bacteria. Microbial imbalances have ramifications throughout the body. You may have heard about the gut-brain connection and how the gut is called the body's second brain. About ninety percent of the serotonin (happiness or good mood chemical messenger) that the brain makes lives in your gut. Oxytocin, also known as the bliss or love hormone, is a chemical messenger that can be found in the gut and binds to interoceptors in the gut. Oxytocin has been observed to improve gut mobility and decrease intestinal inflammation. Unbinding gut fascia can help regulate the flow and balance in the gut, which helps expose the interoceptors. Would you rather roll your gut routinely than pop anti-depressants?

Case study:

Diane, in her later forties, had been dealing with the disabling effects of Hypermobility Syndrome (Ehlers-Danlos Syndrome Type III) for seventeen years. Ehlers-Danlos Hypermobility Syndrome primarily causes musculoskeletal complications like joint dislocation and chronic pain.

Her first episode was shortly after she turned thirty, when she lost the use of both of her arms and had them braced for two years. At her worst point, she told her mom that if she was going to be in that much pain for the rest of her life, she only wanted to live long enough to see her children grown.

Over the past seventeen years, she had accumulated two arm braces, a walking boot, a wheelchair, a cane, and now a brace on her left foot that she had been wearing for the last two and a half years. In this time period, she required two ambulance rides because her back was so tight that she couldn't move her legs or get up off the floor, one ambulance ride because a doctor overdosed her on pain pills and anti-inflammatories that could have killed her, hospitalizations, multiple cortisone shots, years of physical therapy, and most recently back surgery. Medications that had been prescribed to her to deal with the pain included pills to block numb parts of her brain so she didn't feel the pain, pills to numb her nerves, muscle relaxants, and narcotics.

She'd been in physical therapy for her back and foot for two and a half years and she never seemed to get over the "hump" for a full recovery and get rid of the brace on her foot. That's when she decided she needed to try something different and went to Anthony for help after watching The Fascianation Method help many of her friends.

During the first two sessions, focus was on her posture to get her shoulders and head realigned to reduce the strain on her lower back. She had stood improperly for forty-seven years. Postural awareness and mindful posture tweaks shifted the weight in her feet as she walked and put her in a natural position to carry herself. No one had ever addressed her postural deviations before.

Next, Diane used The Fascianation Method to free her tight muscles and further neutralize muscular imbalances in muscles that hadn't worked properly for the last seventeen years. After two sessions, Diane was able to get out of her brace for nearly a week. At an appointment, Diane was asked by her doctor where her foot brace was. Diane explained that she made strides and gained mobility through Anthony's fascial care training. The doctor replied, "Are you going to keep this personal trainer or do you want a refill on your prescription for your pain pills?" That was the first day that her nerve pill dosage was cut in half. She also had the energy and ability to finally go out with her husband night after night! After only a month of self-care, Diane saw her life changing so much that she and her husband renewed their passports and planned a European trip for the following year. Diane stated, "It's time to finally start enjoying life instead of wondering what my next disabling episode is going to be!"

Part 2: Upper Body Rolling

Upper Back (Spinal Erector, trapezius, rhomboids)
These are important posture muscles that you will likely hear crackle when you roll them.

Litmus Test

Before you roll, with your arms to your sides, roll/shrug your shoulders back in a backward circular motion. Repeat after you roll. Compare the difference in smoothness of movement of those muscles. Is it not one of the most fabulous feelings of freedom?

Rolling Technique

You will roll between your spine and your shoulder blades. Place the roller on the mat. Position your mid-back (bra line or the line of the lower chest) onto the roller. Tilt thirty degrees to one side so that you not lying on your spine. Place your hands behind your head. Do not pull your head forward. You are just supporting your head with your hands. Pull your elbows together to bring your shoulder blades away from your spine. This position creates better access to the tissue between your shoulder blades and spine.

Press down through both heels and, while breathing in, push your hips upward. Exhale as you roll the upper back muscles. Roll up toward your shoulders and back down toward the starting point. Switch to the other side of your spine.

Do not roll over spine, ribs, or shoulder blades.

Baby Step Tips

Follow the steps above without lifting your hips. Just lay your upper back muscle on the roller and stay static;

don't roll. Still, with hips on the ground, you may also make short left to right rocking movements. Momentarily lift your hips to reposition your back on the roller. Aim to roll from upper back to mid-back. Don't be discouraged if you are not ready to roll the entire length from upper back to mid-back. Just get used to the sensation of resting your back muscles on the Fascianator for about twenty to thirty seconds. If you are apprehensive, your muscles may contract or tense up versus relax.

If you do not have osteopenia or osteoporosis, another baby step is to roll your upper back without leaning to one side. Be sure to lay only your upper back flat on the Fascianator and keep your elbows down/open instead of pulling them together so that you are not rolling directly over your spine, shoulder blades, ribs, and bony protrusions sticking out from your spine (spinous processes).

Ponder

After you shrug your shoulders, does it feel like your back is looser? Releasing tension around your upper back can help with back, neck, and shoulder pain. Tissue tension in your back and around your spine can free up strain and compression of your nerve roots and your discs.

Upper Latissimus dorsi

These muscles affect your shoulder joint's range of motion as well as your posture.

Litmus Test

Before rolling, test one arm at a time. Rotate your whole arm back in a circular motion as if you are doing a backstroke. Keep your chest and hips facing forward; don't rotate them while making your circular backstroke. Are you able to do this motion smoothly? Is it tight or painful? Do you have to rotate your hips to rotate your arm behind your head? Is the "circular" motion more like a triangle? Take note of your normal range of motion. Is there any clicking sensation? After you roll, repeat the backstroke motion. Can you feel the immediate improvement in the range of motion in your shoulder? Many students have said the crackling in their shoulder joint was resolved after one or two sessions.

Rolling Technique

Lay on your side. Bend the leg that's closest to your mat at a ninety-degree angle and extend the other leg out. Extend your arm up or place it at a ninety-degree angle. Do what's most comfortable. Place the Fascianator in the underarm area. Be sure not to lay on your ribcage. Slowly lean back and forth on the Fascianator. Be sure to relax your neck. Be sure to lean as far back as you can to roll your rotator cuff tendons. Roll as far forward as you can to roll the upper edge of the chest. Do not twist your back. Rotate your hip and spine together.

Ponder

Tight upper back muscles and tight rotator cuff muscles reduce shoulder range of motion. Tight fascia in the underarm (axilla) and chest impede lymphatic drainage away from the upper extremities. Breast cancer survivors who've had axillary lymph node removal often suffer from tight axilla fascia, lymphedema, numbness, and decreased range of motion.

Shoulder

The shoulder has three segments: the front, middle, and the rear segments. When you roll the shoulders you will also roll four of your rotator cuff tendons.

Rolling Technique

Tuck your right arm across your body and, while lying on your right side, place your shoulder on The Fascianator. Bend your knees as you are laying on your side. Rotate your body back, then forward. Be sure to move your pelvis and spine as one unit so that you do not twist your back over your hips. Pay particular attention to the front part of the shoulder muscle. Be sure to avoid any bony protrusions.

Ponder

When you roll the front of your shoulder, your hand on the arm you're rolling may shake. The fascia in your shoulder is connected to your hand. When you roll your shoulders, you are contacting some of the rotator cuff tendons, which often get inflamed, frayed, or ripped when they aren't used enough or are overused. This can be the cause of many cases of shoulder instability.

Chest

Your chest muscles play a large role in posture!

Rolling Technique

In a kneeling position, place the edge of The Fascianator under your clavicle. Turn your arm out while leaning into the edge. Place your opposite hand on the top of The Fascianator. Push in while rolling The Fascianator from the middle of your chest to the outer part of your chest. Roll the roller so that you roll your entire chest muscle. Roll over your breast, too. Fine tune your breast rolling technique/Fascianator positioning to massage all of your breast tissue.

Baby Step Tips

Use less pressure. Using both hands to hold the roller, place the edge of the roller underneath your clavicle. Roll from middle of your chest to the outer part of your chest.

Ponder

Tight chest muscles can pull your shoulders forward, contributing to poor posture and shoulder issues and can impede the flow of lymphatic drainage. There is a lot of lymphatic activity going on in and around your chest. Rolling underneath your clavicle targets the tissue around your thoracic duct, which is the main vessel of the lymphatic system. A rich network of lymphatic vessels runs through your breasts and there are many lymph nodes in your breasts. Since there are no muscle contractions/ pumps in your breasts, take time to roll them to move the lymphatic fluid and reduce calcifications. Take note of any textural changes when you roll over your breasts. Are there fibrous areas? Does your breast become more fibrous during your menstrual cycle? If you are male and reading this, note though it's rare, men also get breast cancer.

Triceps

The back of the upper arm below the shoulder.

Rolling Technique

While laying on one side, place the back of your arm on the Fascianator. Be sure to use your other hand to support your body. With your palm up, turn your thumb out slightly and roll from the base of your elbow up the back of your arm.

Baby Step Tips

Instead of getting down on the floor, place your Fascianator on a counter or table. Sit in a chair or lean over the table and place the back of your upper arm on the roller. With your palm up, turn your thumb out slightly and roll from the base of your elbow up the back of your arm.

Ponder

You may be able to ditch your elbow brace or elbow tendonitis strap if you spend time rolling the soft tissue around your elbow, which would include rolling your triceps.

Bicep

Muscles in the front of arm between your elbow and shoulder joints.

Rolling Technique

While laying on one side, extend your arm out and place the Fascianator on top of your bicep. Be sure to roll both the outside of your bicep and the inside of your bicep. Avoid crossing over your elbow joint.

Ponder

Since your bicep is connected near the groove in your upper arm near your shoulder blade as well as at your forearm near your elbow, when muscles of the biceps are tight, you may feel pain near the front of your elbow (a symptom often referred to as "tennis elbow") and/or pain near the groove in your upper arm (a symptom often referred to as "biceps tendinitis"). You may also feel pain around your thumb.

Forearm Extensors

*Muscles and tendons on top of the forearm that
control and affect movements of the forearm,
wrist, hand, fingers, and thumb.*

Litmus Test

Before rolling each forearm, make a fist with your hands and grip as hard as you can. Take note of the strength of your grip. After you roll each forearm, compare the strength of your grip to your pre-roll grip. You will notice a dramatic improvement in your grip strength.

Rolling Technique

In a kneeling position, place your outer forearm on the Fascianator. Be sure to rotate your forearm outward so your thumb is pointing to the floor to place pressure on the outer part of your forearm, near the outer elbow joint. To fully maximize the technique, be sure to lean your hips and torso outward as well. Take your other hand and place it on top of your forearm and push down on your forearm. Roll down to your wrist and back up, rotating to your outer elbow. Roll all the areas on the topside of your forearm. Lean over to roll the meatiest part of your forearm adjacent to your elbow. Switch sides.

Baby Step Tips

For people who cannot kneel on the ground, this can be done lying on your side with the arm you are rolling extended out to your side and elbow bent up at a ninety-degree angle. It can also be rolled with the Fascianator on a table or counter top.

Ponder

Move each finger up and down and you may see in your forearm that muscles on the top side of your forearm move. Each finger has a corresponding muscle in your forearm that anchors at the elbow. If the muscles on the topside of forearm are tight, pain and stiffness can occur in your fingers (a symptom often referred to as "trigger finger") or pain stiffness can be felt near your elbow (a symptom often referred to as "tennis elbow"). Before using a brace to immobilize your joint or having surgery done to increase your joint range of motion, I recommend giving your tissues some relaxation therapy. Take time to roll the pain away! Rolling will be painful, but remember that the pain and tenderness are messages from your tissues to pay attention to them. The tenderness is pain and tension leaving your body!

Forearm flexors

Muscles and tendons on the underside of the forearm that control and affect movements of the forearm, wrist, hand, fingers, and thumb.

Rolling Technique

In a kneeling position, place forearms on edges of the Fascianator. Press forearms into the edges of The

Fascianator while rolling from near the elbow joint all the way down to the wrists.

Baby Step Tips

For people who cannot kneel on the floor, this technique can be done on a table or countertop.

Ponder

Rolling the underside of the forearm hydrates and loosens the tissue, which can dry and thicken. The stiffness and thickening can place pressure around a nerve that runs down your forearm through the carpal tunnel, which is a passage near the wrist. Before spending thousands of dollars having the fascia in your forearm surgically thinned, try hydrating the tissue and relaxing the pressure on the nerve.

Muscles of Hands

Muscles and tendons of the hands control and affect movements of the palms and fingers.

Rolling Technique

In a kneeling position, place the pinky side of your palm on the edge of the Fascianator. Press your palms into the Fascianator, and roll the muscles of the pinky side of the palm. Slowly move your palms to the edges of the Fascianator, and roll the middle of the palm. Finally, roll the thumb side of your palm over the Fascianator.

Baby Step Tips

For people who cannot kneel on the floor, this technique can be done on a table or countertop. You can also roll while seated on the floor with your feet planted on the floor and your legs bent. Place the Fascianator underneath your knees, and roll your forearms.

Ponder

Repetitive strain of your hands can dehydrate your hand's connective tissue. The stiffness and thickening can make your hand stuck in a partially flexed position (Dupuytren's Contracture). Clients who spend years shelving books in libraries or who grasped dental tools for decades often suffer from hand contractures. One of our clients who suffered from Dupuytren's Contracture was prescribed a brace to wear at night, which made her pain worse. After giving up on immobilizing the hand, our client used The Fascianation Method techniques, which she believed loosened her hand contracture. After measuring the decreased contracture from five degrees to twenty degrees, her doctor counseled her to continue with her fascial therapy and discontinue wearing her brace. Before having the fascia in your hand surgically thinned, take measures to increase your fascia's elasticity; relax and hydrate the tissue of your palms.

Sternocleidomastoid

Front/side of neck

Rolling Technique

Lay on one side of your body and extend your bottom arm out. Tuck the Fascianator all the way into the side of your neck. The Fascianator will be oriented diagonally and the back of the roller will extend behind your ear. Make sure there is no space between your neck and the Fascianator. Hold the long end of The Fascianator down with your other hand. Gently pull your neck into the Fascianator while rotating your chin toward the ceiling. Take a deep breath and exhale while rolling.

Ponder

There are twelve cranial nerves that come down the base of the brain and into the neck. Most of those nerves innervate the face/head. When the muscles and fascia are relaxed on the front and side of the neck as well as behind the ear, pain or numbness felt in the face and head, ringing in the ears and vertigo can be alleviated. Vision can improve. Unexplained dry cough can resolve. The vagus nerve runs from the neck down the chest, along the esophagus, down the diaphragm, and further down the abdominal cavity. The vagus nerve is the second largest nerve and also called the "wanderer" because it branches to various important organs. It innervates parts of the inner ear, voice box, esophagus, heart, lungs, liver, and the upper GI tract. Stimulating the vagus nerve can help reduce stress and anxiety, and counteract a dominant fight or flight response. Recent research has revealed that the vagus nerve can also reset the immune system and regulate the production of pro-inflammatory mediators.

Sub-occipital muscles
Eight muscles at the base of the skull.

Rolling Technique
Find the notch on the base of the skull. Place the Fascianator immediately under the notch. Hold the Fascianator on each end to prevent it from rolling out of position. Pull the base of your skull into the Fascianator while looking left and right.

Ponder
The fascia surrounding the muscles at the base of the skull becomes the dura mater, the sheath that wraps the brain. Relieving the tension of the sub-occipital muscles may also relieve the tension of the tissue that wraps the brain. This tensional release allows fresh oxygenated blood to flow to the head and brain and also allows the drainage of old blood and cellular/metabolic waste from the brain. Dural tension is believed to cause disturbance of the pituitary gland, which regulates the hormonal system. Dural tension is also associated with cerebrospinal fluid disorders that affect the cushioning of the brain and spinal cord. Our clients who suffered from migraines no longer experience chronic migraines. Many are off of their morphine pills for life! From the research that we're reading and years of client feedback, we believe

that other brain issues, syndromes, and even diseases can be mitigated if dural tension is managed. People report clearer vision after Fascianator rolling. The optic tracts at the base of the brain connect to the optic nerves, which are responsible for vision by relaying all visual information including brightness, color, and contrast from the retina to the brain. Rolling the sub-occipital area can stimulate and reduce the tension around the optic conduits.

Neck/Cervical spine

Rolling Technique

Lower the Fascianator down to your cervical spine. Looking straight up at the ceiling, tilt your head back and gently rotate your head to one side of your neck. Stay on one side, rotating back and forth only on that side. Do not put pressure on the very back of your neck. *Stay off the bones of the spinal column.*

Ponder

Have you ever been in a position of having to drive with a stiff neck? Not only rubber-necking causes reckless driving – stiff-necking can be just as dangerous!

Case Study:

Abbie, a retired OB/GYN physician of over thirty years, took Anthony's one-hour Fascianator rolling class twice a week to improve and maintain mobility. After a little over one month, she noticed marked improvement in her flexibility. She could rotate her spine effortlessly to look backwards while driving in reverse. The stiffness in her finger joints from which she had suffered for decades was all gone. This was extremely important because Abbie performed surgeries as an OB/GYN. She found her progress miraculous, but worried that the benefits were due to a strong placebo effect. She had doubts about whether this newfound self-care program would improve her immune system. She was very skeptical of the claims people made about their tendonitis and arthritis disappearing. To Abbie, the technique of myofascial release itself seemed revolutionary, as she felt that there is not much available for the prevention of, or alternative treatment options for, soft tissue injuries. She remained excited about the program and dutifully continued to roll for eight months. The "shocking" results that Abbie gained and attributed to The Fascianator Rolling technique are listed in her own words:

"The arthritis in my hands completely resolved after about one to two months.

I was, for the first time, able to touch my toes while sitting on the floor with my legs extended in front of me. I couldn't even do that in my twenties. Lastly, and the most audacious result: my night vision blindness completely disappeared after about six to eight months of rolling. I drive at night now and I see perfectly. I can see details in very dim lighting without even straining. License plate numbers just jump out at me. I have not done anything different except roll twice a week.

It has been at least a month since this change and even my day vision is more distinct."

Chapter 7:

Cutting Edge

*"Let the lymphatics always receive and discharge naturally.
If so we have no substance detained long enough to
produce fermentation, fever, sickness and death."*

– Andrew Taylor Still (1828–1917),

founder of the field of Osteopathic Medicine

Your body is a sophisticated machine of many synergistic systems. You don't need high technology medicines or devices to maintain your machine. Instead, you need routine environmental care. If you have healthy eating habits and practice The Fascianation Method routinely, you will release natural biochemicals/medicines and avoid unwanted junk festering and fermenting in your body. How often do you brush and floss your teeth? How many teeth do you brush and which surface? I'm sure that you don't only clean the front of your front teeth or the teeth that people see when you smile. To avoid buildup of cavity-causing plaque which can cause gum disease, we brush all of our teeth often. We don't wait for our teeth to fall out or gums to swell before we brush them! We don't have to be bad to get better.

The Fascianator tool is low tech and uncomplicated, but mindfully designed. Don't let the roller's simplicity – no bells or whistles, no knobs or batteries – deter you. This roller was designed with the body in mind. Its diameter and rigidity allow the targeting of certain anatomical structures. It doesn't have bumps or grooves like other rollers. Our intent is for you to feel the knots and inconsistencies in your fascia, not to the feel the bumps and inconsistencies of your roller. We like the high touch and total contact approach. Have a full conversation between you and your new best friend. This methodology, designed to help free up structural imbalances front to back, left to right, top to bottom, is cutting edge in disrupting the immune response that not only causes chronic joint pain, but other inflammatory issues that progress to autoimmune dysfunction. The sophistication is in your fascia so encourage your fascia daily to remain calm and multi-task. It's funny that a tool and methodology so simple is revolutionary and, with respect to current Western medical practice, advanced and cutting edge.

Let's review the immune system, the immune response, and inflammation. The role of our immune system is to protect our bodies from invaders and to repair damaged tissues. Invaders can be viruses, bacteria, yeast, fungus, parasites, allergens, toxins, and cancer cells. Invaders cause infection and toxic or allergic responses. You can imagine that these invaders are all around us twenty-four hours a day, seven days a week. So the immune system is on surveillance 24-7. When a problem is spotted, whether it is gingivitis, hay fever, food allergies, a paper cut, sunburn, or a burned tongue from biting into fresh-baked pizza before the cheese cooled off, an immune response occurs. The response involves chemical messages (inflammatory mediators) and cellular repairmen rushing in to fix the injury or fight the intruder. This is inflammation. You learned that inflammation elicits the pain sensation because of the release of fluid from the blood vessels into the injury site and the release of chemical messages. The type and extent of the response is dependent on the type of intruder and the type of injury. The immune response can get very complicated, especially when there is imbalance of the lymphatic system. So remember ladies, your body is even busier than you remember!

If the body is overwhelmed with chronic healing, stress can further tip the body's imbalance, which causes chronic inflammation, hormonal imbalance, progression to adrenal fatigue and can cause metabolic diseases. There are so many environmental factors that contribute to energy depletion and taxing the body. Our diets, inhalation, skin absorption, unhealthy thoughts, and inadequate rest can introduce toxicity to our bodies. Our bodies respond to these factors in so many different ways that it's hard to know exactly how to beat them. It's hard to pinpoint what causes the trigger pull to autoimmune dysfunction and metabolic diseases. Everyone has a unique genetic story and different level of immunity and tolerance. The best way to disrupt the sustained inflammatory response naturally is to improve the environment by doing daily body housekeeping. Be aware of your aches and pain throughout your body, be proactive in reducing unapparent and low-level inflammation, and hydrate your fascia which lines your organs so that cellular waste and toxins don't embed themselves into that stiff tissue. In autoimmune disease, is the body attacking itself or are the white blood cells targeting the cellular waste, misfolded proteins, or toxins that built up and trapped in stiff and thick tissue?

Corrections in posture can be a catalyst of healing throughout the body. Stiffness and misalignments in the spine cause postural deviations and therefore more muscular and fluid imbalances. When you neutralize the muscular imbalances not only do you have better mobility, you increase blood circulation and drainage of things that cause inflammation, like metabolic waste products and lymphatic waste. Poor lymphatic drainage, in turn, causes fluid buildup and pooling in the body, which creates another inflammatory response. Folks with autoimmune challenges often have stiff, puffy necks, inflamed upper body and forward shoulder posture, which likely impede the flow of lymphatics fluid collected by the thoracic duct and lymphatic duct below the collar bone. Sometimes the puffiness appears to be all over, so people think they've just become fat over time. Our clients with autoimmune conditions have found that our self-care program helps manage the triggers and symptoms of their dysfunction and dis-ease states. Unclogging congestion is key to restrain the inflammation freight train. Keep your blood and your lymphatics flowing. You are your own maintenance superintendent!

Remember those old injuries or intermittent pain sensations? Those can be sources of chronic pain. The most common causes of chronic pain are nerve damage, compression of nerves, and injuries that never heal. The majority of our clients aged forty and above regain proper sensation that was once believed to be nerve damage by freeing the compression caused by tissue thickening around a nerve or nerve root. The thickening is a result of the inflammatory response to persistent strain. An excellent example of damaging thickening around a nerve is carpal tunnel syndrome, which causes pain, tingling, and numbness in the hand and arm. The thickening of the tissue around the median nerve that runs down the arm to the hand compresses the nerve. Immobilizing the wrist might decrease the pressure on the median nerve, but it is also allowing the tissue in the area to become more dry and stiff. If you roll your arm, you can reduce the tension on the median nerve and remodel the fascia and reduce the inflammation. If you've had carpal tunnel surgery, the chances are high that your carpal tunnel issues will return without proper fascial care. About 80% of our clients who've had carpal tunnel surgery complain that their pain came back.

Trigger Point therapy is a chronic pain therapy that targets muscles and the fascia surrounding and penetrating muscles. A trigger point is a small area, a knot within a group of muscle fibers that are in a constant contracted/shortened state. Where there's a trigger point, the muscle fibers don't glide; they are stuck. Trigger points can lead to referred pain; pain not where the knot is, but elsewhere in the body. Trigger point massage stretches the muscle fibers and relaxes the muscle contraction. It increases circulation by clearing the congestion caused by the constant tissue contracture, and it stretches the trigger point's knotted muscle fibers. Trigger point therapy relieves some myofascial dysfunction, but its healing capacity is limited. The Fascianation Method accesses the same stretching mechanisms as trigger point therapy and it provides additional relief because routine whole-body rolling relaxes undesired strain of the body-wide fascial network. It regulates global connective tissue health, not just certain areas around myofascial trigger points.

Pills and injections used to manage injury and chronic pain only treat symptoms. They subdue inflammation and pain but don't address the underlying causes of pain. Reducing inflammation reduces the pain, therefore decreasing the perceived healing time. Decreasing the acute inflammatory response might lead to less pain memory, but if the tension on the tissue persists, inflammation will progress in time. If you keep masking the pain, chances are that you will continue to repeat the activity causing the chronic pain.

People think that a cortisone shot fixes them. Cortisone is a strong anti-inflammatory which might mask pain temporarily, but it shuts down the immune response. Shutting down means that no repairmen are deployed to the trenches. If no one shows up to work, then nothing is fixed. Getting a cortisone shot is like trimming your weeds above the ground. There's no appearance of weeds, but the weeds will still grow. In fact, the roots will grow deeper in the ground. Sometimes people who get steroid injections are worse off than people who don't get injections at all. Infection can ensue in the joint. Cortisone also thins tissue, so you can expect joint's protective cartilage to thin. Ironically, worn cartilage is often the cause of chronic joint pain. For some people, hyaluronic acid joint injections are options for artificial joint lubrication. Multiple doses are required, so each needle puncture is additional damage that causes scar tissue to form at the injection site.

Many of our clients either have joint replacements or are due for replacement surgery. The material used to repair the joint is called a prosthesis and is artificial. Prosthetics are used for disc replacement, hip replacement, knee replacement, shoulder replacement, and, less often, temporomandibular joint (TMJ) replacement. Typically, tissues around the degraded joint are already stiff, dry, and arthritic. Prosthetics can further ruin surrounding tissues because they just don't fit well. Not only do the surrounding tissues remain stiff because nothing is done to hydrate the area for surgery, but new inflammation follows surgery. There are no connective tissue hydration protocols in the rehabilitation regimen. Physical therapy will help strengthen the muscle more than it will relax and lengthen the myofascia. Some prosthetics become surrounded by scar tissue. Sometimes, in the case of disc replacement, it appears that the body tried to push out the prosthesis so the dislocated prosthesis has to be replaced, in which case another tissue-assaulting surgery has to take place. Sometimes an increase in the degree of chronic inflammation in the same area occurs.

Some prostheses are even highly toxic. *The Bleeding Edge* is a horrifying Netflix documentary that discusses the leeching of the toxic heavy metal cobalt in a hip prosthetic. In case you choose to watch the documentary, I will spare you the details, but I must mention that it's believed that the toxicity caused other inflammatory nightmares like Alzheimer's, Parkinson's, and dementia. The Fascianation Method can decrease prolonged joint inflammation, rehydrate the tissue surrounding the prosthesis, and lubricate the joint. In the case of many of our clients, these effects enabled cancellation of joint surgery, even joint replacements. We believe that even bulging discs can be rehydrated and resolved, especially in the cervical spine, if proper corrections in postural deformation are made and lymphatic drainage is increased. You have the control to make the right decisions to improve yourself – don't let things like the wrong health care happen to you. Replacement is a drastic procedure that can improve quality of life or do the opposite. Be aware, do your research and be proactive. If replacement is necessary or was already done, roll around the joint to hydrate the soft tissues of and surrounding the joint before and after the surgery.

Stiffness or weakness of the muscles in the abdominal region can prevent proper muscle activation for breathing efficiency. Intercostal muscles help the diaphragm lift the ribcage so that the lungs can expand. If the intercostal muscles aren't correctly firing, muscles in the neck are recruited to help out. What if the neck muscles aren't properly activated to help out? When spinal and muscle imbalances are neutralized, upper body posture is corrected, and breathing is improved. Even asthma can be managed using The Fascianation Method. Optimal breathing helps the body stay balanced and keep energy levels up. Eliminating dis-ease is the first step in fighting progression to disease! Even better news is that, with the proper self-care that you'll continue to read about in Chapter 8, disease can be reversible!

If I were in a bad car accident or in need of emergency care for acute trauma such as an appendix rupture or bypass surgery, then I would welcome the marvels of modern medicine. If I am ripped or cut open, I'll take the drugs! I played Wonder Woman once, bearing my second child without pain management drugs, drips, or injections, and that alone was enough birth control for me! There are times when surgery and medication are very appropriate and necessary. I don't believe that commuting to work, working at the office every day, jogging, swimming, or gardening should warrant habitual pill popping, diagnostic imaging, or going under the knife for exploratory or therapeutic surgery. Activities that involve repetitive strain necessitate self-care and shouldn't require therapy.

Asthma Case Study

Sally, in her late forties, had had allergies since infancy and she had her first asthma attack at eighteen months old. She had been a lifetime asthma sufferer. She had "remodeled" lungs; structural changes/fibrosis in the airway due to chronic inflammation. On a great day, Sally could breathe about seventy percent of her lung volume capacity. She took low dosage asthma medication and increased her lung health with healthy eating habits and exercised three to five days a week. Still, she also took supplements or medication to really open and increase her lung capacity. She could never do diaphragmatic breathing. After trying The Fascianation Method, she felt her lungs open up and truly felt that a restriction had "let go" in her diaphragm area. She continues to roll twice a week and her lungs have sustained lung volume (even after catching a mild flu/cough). She no longer takes supplements or medication for her lungs to work efficiently.

Cancer

When the immune system is already taxed, the accumulation of inflammatory molecules in a stiff, congested, and stagnant environment causes a shift in pH balance. The environment can become very acidic, which adds to the recipe of cell transformation. These conditions can cause happy, normal cells in the area to be recruited to inflammatory situations. If the cells are freed from the mechanically stressed environment, the transformation to cancer cells can be controlled. If tissue and matrix strain persist, inflammation and stagnation get worse, oxygen availability decreases, pH levels drop, and the genetic predispositions to cancer are switched on. The environment is too stressed to fix random DNA mutations. The environment is not only pro-fibrotic, but pro-cancer. My own tissue culture experiments have demonstrated that cancer thrives in acidic and hypoxic microenvironments. Activities like exercise that increase blood circulation and lymphatic drainage are vital to keeping cancer at bay. The Fascianation Method not only increases circulation and mechanically pumps the lymphatics for drainage, it induces the right tensional forces on the tissues to shift the stressed environment to a more balanced state.

Dr. Helen Langevin, Director of the Osher Center for Integrative Medicine at Harvard Medical School and Brigham and Women's Hospital conducted a mouse model study in which manual stretching reduced experimentally induced inflammation. Dr. Langevin's studies suggest that stretching can control inflammation and support immune cells that kill cancer cells. Stretching can be an essential component of cancer treatment and prevention. A little stretching goes a long way!

In a nutshell, The Fascianation Method can help you keep a neutral environment that may prevent random mutations and genetic dispositions from turning cancer switches on.

Blood Cancer and Amyloidosis Case Study:

Pat was diagnosed with multiple myeloma (MM) complicated with amyloidosis. MM is a cancer of plasma cells and amyloidosis simply defined as a buildup of excess proteins in the body, which can deposit in any organ, the nervous system, gastrointestinal tract, etc. Both are considered treatable but generally incurable.

Pat's treatment was weekly chemotherapy for three months, which was an hour of an IV chemotherapy cocktail followed by a shot in the belly and oral chemotherapy pills. The therapy was all in preparation for the eventual stem cell transplant that she underwent at the Mayo Clinic in Rochester, Minnesota a few months later. Over a total of seven weeks and about four thousand miles away from her home, Pat met with various doctors, took numerous tests, had a couple of surgeries, took nutrition classes and caregiver classes for her husband, underwent stem cell collection, and had two days of intense chemotherapy.

Pat went back to work weeks later. Pat also suffered from carpal tunnel and "hardening" of arteries that caused her heart to race even when sitting still. After three months of recovery, Pat incorporated The Fascianation Method of self-care into her healthcare regimen to keep all the fluids moving in her body, which she hoped would prevent the cancer and amyloidosis from recurring. Two years later and still rolling, the doctors checked for deposits in Pat's liver and routinely checked for swelling in her ankles, lymph nodes, tongue, etc. Pat's blood is healthy and she is cancer-free.

Chapter 8:
Lifestyle Changes

"All life is an experiment.
The more experiments you make, the better."
–Ralph Waldo Emerson

Imagine all of the possible inflammatory events currently going on in your body. Add chronic psychological stress, because scientists have determined that mental stress can cause a depressed immune function. Now add sub-optimal nutrition (not enough nutrients and antioxidants from "rainbow food," a.k.a. green, purple, red, yellow, orange vegetables; too much processed food; too much sugar; chemically tainted food). Is it any wonder why sometimes, even with enough sleep, your body and/or mind is still sluggish? Can you see why folks in tip-top shape or those who are relatively healthy hit a certain age and their bodies really start rebelling against them and "falling apart?"

You now understand that many factors that can cause pain to persist or come back. These are physical factors and psychological factors that have the common theme of stress and tension. You know that some of the fascial network's talent is to receive and forward information to regulate homeostasis and to keep the body's architecture balanced. When tension and stress make your fascia dry and stiff, the repairmen are deployed to help bring balance to the area. They may even mitigate pain. Being chronic pain free is a lifestyle that equips the team of security guards, dispatchers, repairmen, and cleanup crew inside of your body to work in harmony.

Once the body is freed from nagging fascial restrictions, the muscles have to be retrained again. Your body will be loosened in a way that it has never relaxed before. Rolling is not the only self-care that you should be doing. The body needs a balance of tension and looseness. Before going back to play full speed ahead, don't be overzealous. Too much looseness results in instability. Too much tension results in muscular imbalances. What needs to be incorporated in the pain free living regimen is exercise to re-engage the muscles to learn how the stabilize the newly loosened joint. Pretend you are the puppet and you are also the puppet master. To prevent imbalances, you have to make sure that you maintain a sufficient amount of muscle strength and stabilization as you continue to roll out your soft tissue. Exercises that you can do are bodyweight-only exercises. You do not want to add additional resistance at this point. You also want to execute the movements deliberately and slowly. Do squats or safely sit back in a chair firing your leg muscles and get back up. You can also do leg lunges. You can do pushups off of your wall, kitchen counter, or chair. Pushups on your knees are fine, too. The exercises are simple movements to engage your muscles after you loosen them up. Remember that more is not always better. Performing a slow and controlled set of four to twelve repetitions of these exercises twice a week is good.

I talk about hydration so much and I'll say it again! Remember that fascia is primarily composed of water and it stores one-fourth of our body's water. On average, a person has about forty pounds of fascia in them. We should drink plenty of water – H_2O, meaning plain old boring water, versus sugary drinks or liquids that are diuretics like coffee or tea, which cause us to lose water through frequent urination. For every cup of diuretic, drink double that volume in water and to replenish what you'll lose from the diuretic. A simple daily water intake guideline that I suggest is to take your body weight in pounds and divide that value by two. That is the *minimum* amount of water in ounces that you should strive to drink daily. For example, if I weight one hundred pounds, then I should drink fifty ounces of water daily. One hundred divided by two equals fifty. If you are someone who is always warm or perspires or sweats a lot, you should drink even more water. When you are on your period you lose more water volume than usual, so increase your water intake during your special time.

After rewiring your tensional network with The Fascianation Method, engage in other activities that support fascial health. Movement helps to lubricate your joints. Your movement practice doesn't have to be intense. You also don't want to be overzealous and go straight into Spartan Race mode. Start slow, taking note of your new abilities. Gradually build up your pace, duration, and weight (for resistance training). A leisurely stroll with a mindful, deliberate gait is a great way to engage your lengthened muscles. Avoid letting your feet drag; plant your heel and roll to the ball of your foot, then off of your toes. The rolling action makes your gait more elastic. Swing your arms forward and back to engage your chest and back muscles and to increase your heart rate. Don't forget to drink water while you're strolling!

The best activities are ones that incorporate multi-directional and spiraling movement. Think about your daily movement. Do you move like an old school robot where your movements take place in one plane at a time? "Either/or" repetitive movement is where you either move forward, backward, pivot left, or pivot right, up or down. Smooth, twisting, and rotating movement is much better for the body. Good movement practices include Fascial Fitness, yoga, Tai Chi, and Pilates. These practices will help you develop an intimate awareness of your fascia and will enhance whole person health to mitigate chronic pain. If you practice the movements mindfully, deliberately, and in moderation, you should become more injury resistant and balanced. You should also find that moving helps manage your mental stress level. In your journaling, take note of how your movement practice makes you feel, mentally and physically.

Fascial Fitness® was developed based upon the research of Rolfer practitioner and pioneering fascia researcher Dr. Robert Schleip. Dr. Schleip's wife, Divo Gitta Müller, a Somatic Experience practitioner, played a key role in the practical development of the movement program. Some of the movements stem from dance technique, incorporating low impact bouncing and spinal undulations. Another training movement is emulating a wood chop arm swing (without the ax), using an elastic, smooth pendulum swing. Foam rolling myofascial release is also an element of the Fascial Fitness program. The training elements preserve and enhance fascia's elasticity and springiness. You will release, stretch, and have better elastic movement.

Yoga can help develop muscle tone and flexibility as well as breathing and mental focusing techniques. There are about fourteen types of traditional yoga and about thirty types of modern-day yoga practices. Some schools of yoga focus on philosophy and meditation versus positions and techniques. Some offer a good combination of all of those elements and more. Some classes are very structured, possibly intense and others are free-flowing, more relaxed in structure and in poses. Since a wide array of yoga styles exist, you will want to explore and experiment to see which practice and instructors suit you best. After using your Fascianator to "thaw" your tissues, I recommend that you try Yin Yoga, which is a slow-paced style of yoga that promotes soft tissue rehydration, blood and fluid balance, and therefore restoration. I also recommend diversifying your movement practice, if possible. Another type of yoga that I recommend that will kill two birds with one stone, both cardiovascular and muscular (resistance) training, is Vinyasa, also called Ashtanga. Vinyasa is a fast-paced series of postures or asanas that focuses on the flow *between* movements, rather than individual poses. Many of our clients with fibromyalgia feel great benefit doing Bikram or "hot" yoga.

Tai chi is a type of Chinese internal martial art that was originally developed for self-defense and has evolved into a very graceful movement practice. In Tai chi, you flow into various postures without pause, which provides balance, breathing, mindfulness, and general fitness training.

Pilates is a movement system that was developed by Joseph Pilates. There are various forms of Pilates training. Some Pilates training is all mat-based work where you use your own bodyweight to create resistance. There is another type of Pilates training that uses the Reformer machine. The Reformer is a sliding platform in which you kneel, sit, stand, or lie. The user hangs on to handles that are attached to a cable-pulley to push or pull your body with added resistance. This requires focused and controlled movement. There is a lot of muscle stabilization involved. Pilates training focuses on the core musculature. Many people believe the core to be just the abdominal muscles. Muscle groups that support the body's core are in the abdomen, lower back, hips, and butt. Movement stems from the core, so Pilates is great balance, flexibility, and strength training.

All of the movement practices that I mentioned are great ways for light/bodyweight resistance training and, they are wonderful ways of increasing blood, lymphatic, and energy flow. I reiterate that one can be overzealous with any exercise. When learning new techniques, take it slow in the beginning to understand your limitations and always be mindful of your movements.

In Chapter 4, I discussed mental housekeeping techniques to help you stay positive and mentally aligned. It's important to set your day up right to reinforce the positive mindset that not only keeps you motivated, but also helps you manage stress. Another stress management tool that I suggest is diffusion of essential oils. Essential oils are safe, volatile oils distilled from the most fragrant part of plants (seeds, bark, leaves, stems, roots, flowers, and fruit). Since the oils are volatile, their aromas affect the limbic lobe or emotional center of the brain and they penetrate the blood brain barrier unlike medications. They can elicit positive neurological, emotional, and behavioral effects. There are about 188 references to essential oils in the Bible so essential oils have been counted on well before multilevel marketing commissions existed. I use these one hundred percent therapeutic grade essential oils for calming effects: lavender, ylang ylang, spruce, spearmint, frankincense, bergamot, and sage.

Lavender (Lavandula angustifolia) is one of my favorites to diffuse before I go to bed. It has been documented to help with anxiety and sleep disturbances. Various university research studies reveal that inhalation of lavender modulate brain wave activity and suggest benefits like heightened relaxation, reduced depression, and reduced mental stress. There are other added benefits of lavender. Topical application of lavender oil has been associated with external wound healing. Research shows that lavender helps keep the inflammatory response balanced so that the myofibroblast repairmen lay down collagen but are not allowed to work overtime.

Ylang ylang (Cananga odorata) is another oil that I diffuse alone and sometimes blend with other known anti-inflammatory oils like lavender and lemon. It is known to filter out negative energy, combat anger, balance male-female energy, enhance spiritual attunement, and also dilate blood vessels. In Indonesia flowers Ylang ylang are spread on the bed of newly wed couples. Another interesting fact about Ylang Ylang is that it is widely used in floral-themed perfumes like Chanel No. 5.

Spruce (there are several species of plants used for oils) has an earthy scent and is very calming and grounding. The sweet tree scent treats me to a virtual escape frolicking in nature. Native Americans used spruce for both mind and body harmony. Spruce is well-documented to have positive effects on our multiple body systems, including our endocrine, respiratory, nervous, and immune systems.

Spearmint (Mentha spicata) opens and releases emotional blocks, bringing about a feeling of balance. It's not as strong as peppermint so it has more of a relaxing effect than invigorating effect. It also has anti-inflammatory properties and has been used in ancient times for digestive issues.

Frankincense (Boswellia carterii) has been used for thousands of years for ceremonies and medicine for many countries. Frankincense has been mentioned in one of the oldest known medical records of the Ancient Egyptians. It's known to uplift spirits, increase spiritual awareness, promote meditation, stimulate the immune system, and have anti-inflammatory properties.

Bergamot (Citrus aurantium bergamia) is used for anxiety, hormonal fluctuations, and depression. Bergamot gives Earl Grey tea its distinctive flavor and is a key component in many colognes.

Sage (Salvia officinalis) was called the sacred herb by ancient Romans. Sage strengthens vital centers of the body by balancing the second/pelvic chakra, where negative emotions from denial and abuse are stored. It combats anxiety and mental fatigue.

I also use essential oil blends as much as possible in place of over-the-counter drugstore cold, allergy, bloating, gas, upset stomach, infection, cough, inflammation, and bug repellent remedies. After spending a lot of time in the lab working with chemicals, I've noticed I have developed a higher sensitivity to vapors of off the shelf chemicals like adhesives, bleach, ammonia, other household cleaners. I prefer to use nature's medicine, healthy foods and essential oils over chemically synthesized drugs. Especially as we age, it's critical to be wary of the chemical toxins that buildup in our tissues. Accumulation of junk in our tissues can cause chronic issues years down the road.

An anti-inflammatory lifestyle, would, of course, involve eating non-inflammatory foods. Eating whole, unprocessed foods decreases the level of inflammation in your body. Whole foods don't have a nutrition label on them. They are foods without added preservatives such as meat, fish, eggs, fresh fruits, raw nuts, and vegetables.

Avoid foods that cause inflammation. As mentioned before, different people have different sensitivities to foods and substances. Almost all convenience foods, meaning pre-packaged (which often contain preservatives and stabilizers), processed, and refined foods cause inflammation. The inflammation can be low grade, so people used to eating these types of foods typically don't notice an inflammatory effect. Cumulatively, the effects of low-grade inflammation could manifest in a physical issue over time. If you are in the middle of an inflammation nightmare and having autoimmune dysfunction, low-grade inflammation might take your system to the next level of "healing" chaos. Your body can be in such an inflamed state it can lose the ability to discern who's a good worker in your body and who's a bad worker. Any tissue that is irritated by toxin accumulation or fermentation of old waste can become a target for immune attack.

More obvious inflammatory foods are fruits and vegetables that were grown around glyphosate, the harmful chemical component found in the herbicide RoundUp. If you want to really be on the safe, anti-inflammatory side you should only buy organic fruits, vegetables, and grains with a reputable source. Some farmers grow organically but do not have the funding to certify their facilities as organic growers. Shop around and look for safe produce from well-respected environmentally-conscious sources. Better yet, you might find it gratifying and therapeutic to grow your own produce! I grow a lot of my own vegetables with a Tower Garden, a low maintenance aeroponic growing system. I spent a few years testing harsh chemicals that were used as pesticides. I witnessed firsthand the negative effect of pesticides on my cell cultures.

If you're a barbecue fan, I have bad news for you. Charred and seared meats cause inflammation. The blackened char contains two types of chemicals that cause cancer in animal studies.

If you want to use a methodical approach to determine what foods might not be agreeable to your gut or trigger an immune response, try an elimination diet. Inflammatory symptoms can be chronic joint pain, headaches, abdominal bloating, gas, acid reflux, skin rash, or lethargy. The GODS elimination can start with avoiding G=gluten, O=oils, D=dairy, and S=sugar. I know, you see what GODS stands for and you're thinking, "Oh GODS, so what can I eat and actually enjoy?" I've been there and found it very hard to get used to the GODS elimination diet if you are at a loss for food options. Refer to Pinterest for a plethora of elimination guidelines and options. You may have to start cooking every meal yourself and that can be very empowering. How badly do you want to find out your triggers? It usually takes about three to six weeks of elimination diet diligence to determine your food sensitivities.

Gluten is in a lot of grains, breads, wheat products, and noodles, and you'll find it in a lot of sauces. Although you may not be highly sensitive to gluten, you may find out that you have more energy if you eliminate it from your diet. Some people have reactions to products that have ingredients that have been genetically modified. In addition to looking for organically grown and certified foods, look for foods that have non-GMO ingredients.

Since there is a lot of conflicting information reported on which oils are bad, consume oils in moderation. The top four oils that I see are always or most often characterized as good oils are olive oil, grapeseed oil, avocado oil, and coconut oil. What's of interest in oil is the ratio of omega-6 fatty acids to omega-3 fatty acids. Omega-6 is known to be more inflammatory than omega-3, so choosing oils with more omega-3 fatty acids is ideal in an anti-inflammatory diet. I take a tablespoon of lemon flavored cod liver oil once daily to get a good dose of omega-3 fatty acids.

Cow dairy products, even yogurt, and especially ice cream and cheese are pro-inflammatory for many people with allergies or metabolic disease. You can try goat dairy as a substitute. Goat milk has less of an inflammatory effect. If you like drinking milk, try drinking almond milk or soy milk.

Excess sugar intake, especially refined sugar is bad for our tissues. Sugar accumulation can cause glycation, which is the strong bonding of a sugar molecule to a protein molecule. The accumulation of dietary sugar in tissues causes inflammation and tissue aging. Sugar can get stuck in diabetics' blood vessels which damage vessels. Glycation changes viscosity between fascial layers, which disrupts the gliding between fascial layers and can create fascial density changes that can lead to chronic pain. Good alternative sweeteners are natural honey, agave, coconut oil, and stevia. I even bake gluten-free cookies with agave, honey, and coconut oil.

After eliminating GODS, you can slowly add back foods from one category at a time to investigate what you might be allergic to.

Earlier I mentioned rainbow vegetables. You've probably heard that the vegetables that are the most colorful have the most nutrients and antioxidants in them. One of my favorite rainbow vegetables with high anti-inflammatory properties is broccoli. The stalks are just as nutritious as the florets. Dark leafy greens like kale and spinach are also some of my favorite high vitamin and mineral anti-inflammatory veggies. Purple cabbage is another favorite rainbow vegetable. While these vegetables can be eaten raw, if you're not used to eating lots of raw vegetables, I suggest that you break down the leaves in a powerful blender or better yet, sauté or blanch the leaves for quicker gut absorption.

Unfortunately, some of those vegetables cause inflammation in people. There is a group of vegetables called nightshade vegetables that many people are allergic to. Some people also have inflammatory issues with vegetables that have lectins in them. Lectins are a type of protein that the body can't break down easily. Lectins can be found in the vegetable skin and seeds. If you determine that certain fruits or vegetables cause inflammation, try peeling the skin and removing the seeds. One way of helping to break down lectins is to cook the vegetables in order to destroy the lectin in its form that causes inflammation.

For many people, modulating the body's innate antioxidant system with a ketogenic diet helps to reduce chronic inflammation. In a ketogenic diet, ketones derived from fats are used for energy instead of carbs. Ketogenic foods are fish, shellfish, low carbohydrate vegetables and fruits, cheese, red meat and poultry, eggs, yogurt, and nuts. Beware that there are hardcore ketogenic diet programs that are not healthy for all people for long-term nutrition. They can make the body very sick by making the body go into the metabolic state of ketoacidosis. During ketoacidosis, high levels of ketones build up to dangerous levels in individuals with low insulin levels. This can cause acidic blood pH and calcium and magnesium depletion from the bones to buffer the low blood pH.

So, we talked about food – now let's talk about the elimination of all the waste your body can't use. How do you improve elimination? Remember that The Fascianation Method will help mechanically move the buildup of waste in your intestines and help your bowel movement quality. Also, improved physical activity, hydration, and fiber uptake you to urinate and sweat more regularly. Those things I mentioned are housekeeping chores that affect inflammation and the balance and flow of our bodies. I have clients who not only have to learn how to exercise more but hate drinking water because they don't like to pee. There are water trackers on phone apps and fitness trackers; I wonder if there are pee trackers. Some of my clients don't seem to pee as much as they should be based upon how much they report they drink. Hmmmmmm… I sense an imbalance like a bladder infection in the horizon.

Use other tools like a gua sha scraper to improve circulation, reduce soft tissue tension, and stimulate an immune response. In Chinese, gua refers to the scraping or scratching of the skin. Sha refers to the rash, blood vessel disruption, or redness that appears after scraping. The gua sha scraper is smooth-edged. A lotion or oil lubricant can be applied to the skin before the scraper is pressed into the skin and slow unidirectional strokes are used to cause enough tissue trauma to elicit an immune response. The controlled tissue damage leads to the wound healing process. It can even break down scar tissue. The gua sha tool can be used on tight areas where the Fascianator doesn't "floss" like in between the ribs, in between the finger and toe articulations, and around and on top of your head. The gua sha tool can be used around the face using less pressure to stimulate tissue hydration and relieve tension.

Even if you have been using The Fascianation Method regularly to maintain your tissue integrity and maintain musculoskeletal balance, you might once in a blue moon have an accidental strain or pull after engaging in a new activity or dramatically increasing the intensity of physical activity. Remember when I was stuck in the ocean hanging onto my canoe and contending with the current much longer than expected? The following day I felt great and grateful! Hey, I had both of my feet planted on soil and was no longer shark bait! Feeling like a seasoned fighter and having bruises that surfaced in various areas, I did a celebratory boot camp style workout without thinking about how overworked my bad shoulder, chest, and neck were from the previous day. That night I fell asleep on the couch in a contorted position and the following morning my right upper torso was out of whack. I felt a rib may have been out of place. I Fascianator rolled and felt much better, but as the day progressed I had some mobility challenges. It was dangerous for me to drive because I couldn't turn my neck to look over my right shoulder. I tried making an appointment to see whoever could see me first – my chiropractor or my acupuncturist, who also does fascial release. Unfortunately, that week I couldn't see any of my practitioners, so I continued to roll, stretch, and rest my body. After about two weeks of rolling, stretching, and resting, my aches and pains disappeared. I continue my toe to head soft tissue care regimen to keep unwinding old kinks and new kinks.

Once in a while you may have to see a chiropractor, bodyworker, or acupuncturist to work on fascial restrictions immediately or to fix your ribs or spine that are misaligned. Especially in the case of an injury or accident, if you discuss the nature of your accident and explain how you were injured, a chiropractor or a bodyworker trained in soft tissue release may be able to determine the specific areas that need to be worked on. They are trained to see and/or palpate areas that need to be adjusted/relaxed. Remember that the pain doesn't tell us exactly where the fascial distortions causing the pain may be.

Chapter 9:

Roadblocks or Bumps in The Road

"Don't think. FEEL. It's like a finger pointing at the moon. Do not concentrate on the finger or you will miss all the heavenly glory."
– Bruce Lee

During your chronic pain journey, you will encounter "life happens" events and distractions that will interfere with your momentum and will appear as reasons to take a detour from your destination to Pain Free Living. Remember that this journey is a "new you" journey. It's all about you and your goal. Your goal may be tough, but you have achieved tough goals in the past. You *can* achieve your health goal as long as you believe in your goal. Your goal is waiting for you. Show up and do not quit on yourself.

I need not remind you that life isn't always fair and you only get so many chances. Take advantage of today. Don't think about your pain. Recognize it, feel it, and focus on blessings and healing. Take the information that you have read so far and put it into action! Here are some strategies for you to use when "life happens," especially when "crap happens," and you feel like you need to prioritize other things besides your well-being. You have to live in your body, not just in your brain.

1. Are you giving up before giving it a chance? You didn't have chronic pain overnight, so don't expect to get rid of the pain quickly. Give yourself one to three months of consistent rolling before you make any efficacy judgments. Give your body time to adjust. Past clients of ours who have only rolled sporadically realized that the changes truly happen after they are consistent in showing up to the appointments they've made with themselves. Be your own leader. Let your decisions control the repair crews in your body; don't let them control you.

2. Re-evaluate: Identify the reasons for your lapse in practicing your whole body rolling at least twice a week.

3. Identify what needs to be done/changed in order for you to progress toward action again. Do you need to reschedule your calendar or someone else's to make time for yourself? Do you need to change your bed or wake time? There will always be a valid

reason for you to justify taking a break from your practice. Making the situational adjustment may not be easy, but it is essential to stay in the driver's seat with the same GPS guide.

4. Revisit your support systems. Reestablish the relationships that you had with the people who were excited and encouraging of your goal to attain chronic pain free living. You've read this far. We support you and we believe in you! Please contact us and we'll chat.

These are some of the excuses that clients have given us in the past:

"I Don't Have Time"

If you think you don't have time to roll, don't overthink. After your morning mindset ritual or before bed, pick up your Fascianator, grab your instructions, follow the MP4 video, pop in the DVD, and just start rolling. You owe it to yourself to run through the exercise at least once a day to see how your body responds. Grant yourself a break if you need. No judgment. Don't berate yourself for not being able to complete the whole hour of rolling. If you are a perfectionist, try to let go of the perfectionist mindset. Your body is not perfect, so don't expect your mind-body to perform perfectly. This is an exploration process.

Start with baby steps again. Upon waking up, set a timer for six minutes to do the early morning ritual. Set the timer for fifteen minutes and roll for fifteen minutes.

Before going to bed, set the timer for fifteen minutes and roll again.

Choose one problem area and roll to address that area. Repeat every day for two weeks then increase your rolling time and effort.

Loving yourself can be an everlasting journey because circumstances change. Deliver on your commitments to yourself. Show up!

"I Don't Have Space"

While it would be nice to have a dedicated space to roll, you don't need a Zen fountain beside your yoga mat to have the serenity to ensure tensional release. If you can lay on the floor, you have space. If you belong to a gym or can find a community space, bring your Fascianator to the gym and roll there. If you are reading this book, you are due to find space to take care of *you* again. The more you roll, the more benefit you'll feel, and the more space you are creating in your mind and body to have more peace. Isn't peace the most serene space?

"Body Going Back to Old Ways of Pain"

Once you start feeling better, don't think that that's the end of your pains. You may no longer have chronic pain, but you may still feel stiffness at times. If you continue the same activities or sedentary pattern, your soft tissue and fascia will want to revert to their old tensional patterns. The pain wants to come back, but you have to keep telling your pain that there's no home for it. Mechanisms for change take time. You have to be patient. Give it at least a couple of months. You didn't develop what's given you chronic pain overnight and you will not be able to unwind your fascia overnight. Be hopeful and remember that humans have great potential for change or plasticity!

"Other People Don't Like the New Me"

You've probably shared your progress with other people out of excitement for yourself and for them to learn a powerful new process of self-care. Some hop on your bandwagon and some think you are out of your mind, wasting your time, or selfish. Do not let other people's negativity, maybe jealousy, or whatever their issue is with themselves discourage you or affect your success. The new you will have more spirit and joy. You will have new independence that other people will admire and wish they had for themselves, but they haven't created space within them to delve into the unfamiliar. It takes courage to love and it takes even more courage to love yourself enough to not put your health into someone else's hands.

We have never come across this situation, but in case you are an outlier, if you have done the two times per week whole body rolling in earnest for at least six months, and you feel pain that is chronic, see your physician, a functional medicine doctor, a reputable holistic professional such as a licensed acupuncturist, bodyworker (myofascial release practitioner, structural integrationist, or Rolfer) and/or reputable chiropractor. You can also contact us. We can help you troubleshoot. You may want to reevaluate your lifestyle and explore factors such as water intake, nutrition, heavy metals toxicity, parasite infection, movement patterns such as overuse/repetitive stress, thought patterns, and quality of sleep.

Chapter 10:

Restore, Rebalance, Reclaim

"Arise! For this matter is your responsibility but we will be with you. Be courageous and act."

– Ezra 10:4

"Give away your life; you'll find life given back, but not merely given back - given back with bonus and blessing. Giving, not getting, is the way. Generosity begets generosity."

– Luke 6:37-38

By choosing to read this book, you were chosen to spread and grow our fascial care movement. It is not by mistake or luck that we are speaking to you. Your curiosity, your open-mindedness, and your courage to explore beyond the myopic focus of the obsolete medical institution paradigm call you to help me empower other women. Instead of rehabilitating, let's simultaneously and proactively pre-habilitate. This process is not discriminatory and applies to everyone; young and old, female and male, one-legged, and used by people with paralysis of both legs. Although the case studies that we presented are all female, we have opened our doors and welcome all walks of life to our workshops. Interestingly, at our group workshops, we have about a 10% male attendance rate. Why?

We believe it's because women are the nurturers and in their hearts, they want to be well so that they can continue taking care of other people, whether it be at home, work, school, church, social clubs, or all the above. Are you still a frequent multi-tasker even after much research has shown that multi-tasking is not good for the average person's brain? You may argue that you are not the average person! The average person remains disempowered and is relegated to further suffering. In our movement, we help restore power back to individuals. We teach people to have a new awareness of their own minds and bodies. This new awareness supports a holistic approach to minimizing toxic influences in our bodies, thoughts, and emotions. We have reached a time of exciting universal shifting. Much needed paradigm shifts are crucial now to restore and reduce global dissonance. Please harness your power. Take advantage of your curiosity to seek better information and care for yourself today. Feel the difference in our chronic pain relief program and share your results with others, especially women who are selfless and practically give away their lives while giving life to their tribes. You never know whose life you might save by choosing to act. It might be your own.

Tell women who fit the shoes that the ball is in their court. Rolling will give them more energy and strength to pull through hopelessness. Tell women who you recognize as having chronic pain but who haven't yet accepted the "chronic pain" label themselves about this book. Self-awareness is the key to healing. Typically people with an auto-immune condition like Hashimoto's Disease or lupus have chronic pain and high pain thresholds. Their bodies are equipped to manage or stop chronic pain even if they have been told otherwise. They may have been told that their condition is permanent or that their condition can only be monitored and their symptoms only treated. We have reduced the chronic pain and have seen positive blood chemistry changes in our clients with Hashimoto's and lupus. The reality is that with faith and determined effort, what we thought were degenerative disease processes have the potential to be reversed.

If you are a male who has read this far, congratulations on being one of the special ones! You are intuitive and wise. You can follow the same methodology to take the healing power back in your own hands. Share with others what you have learned about stopping chronic pain now without pills, injections, and surgery.

Don't wait for a more convenient situation. Don't wait to act until you create more space to reprogram your system. As we wrap up writing this book, we learned that our high school classmate, a lupus warrior unexpectedly passed away while fighting kidney disease. She was a beloved mother, friend, and family day care owner with a zeal for life, a gentle heart of gold, a kind soul. Three days ago, we announced the date of our book release and just yesterday this former classmate messaged us that she needed to get a copy of our book. We're so sad that we didn't get the information in our book out to her sooner. Sometimes just one or two months can change someone's healing trajectory. Take action now to practice alternative forms of healing. Take care of yourself as dearly as you take care of the people you love and serve.

The reality is that you can revitalize, rejuvenate, restore, rebalance, reclaim, reinvent, and realize our potential and purpose again. You have another shot! You can reactivate your gym membership, return to your dance classes, reignite your passions by reacquainting yourself with your fascia. Reconnect!

Remember Val from Chapter 1 who had fibromyalgia, was losing motivation and beginning to feel like life was all downhill after age 52? In the past five years, Val fulfilled her education dream by finishing her bachelor's degree and pursuing even higher education. She obtained her master's degree in education, earned a graduate certificate in online learning and teaching, and is currently working on her Ph.D. Val tells me that her fascia is still her best friend!

Further Reading

If you would like to learn more about the fascinating world of fascia, please check out the following references that I used to write this book;

1. Langevin, H. et al., (2018 May 18), *Stretching Reduces Tumor Growth in a Mouse Breast Cancer Model*, retrieved from http://www.Nature.com
2. Lesondak, David, *Fascia What it is and Why it Matters*, Handspring Publishing Ltd, 20176.
3. Oschman, James, L., *Energy Medicine, Elsevier Ltd., 2016.*
4. Rolf, Ida, *Rolfing: Reestablishing the Natural Alignment and Structural Integration of the Human Body for Vitality and Well Being*, Healing Arts Press, 1989.
5. Schleip, Robert; Findley, Thomas; Chaitow, Leon; Huijing, Peter, *Fascia: The Tensional Network of the Human Body*, Elsevier Ltd., 2012.

Acknowledgments

Thank you, Mom and Dad, for your unconditional love, faith, and support for the things that we do that you may not understand at first but you ultimately honor.

Thank you, Dr. Shanaz Dairkee, for being such an inspiring, trusting teacher and role model. The day that you told said "people only get so many chances" was the day that my tenacity shot up exponentially.

Thank you to the Morgan James Publishing team: Special thanks to David Hancock, CEO & Founder for believing in us and our message. To our Author Relations Manager, Tiffany Gibson, thanks for your compassion, going above and beyond and making the process seamless and easy. Many more thanks to everyone else, but especially Jim Howard, Bethany Marshall, and Nickcole Watkins.

Thank you, Angela Lauria. Writing this book has been a very introspective process, much harder than we thought. Your brilliance created an amazing program that brings together many inspiring leaders like yourself. Your guidance and coaching are invaluable to infinity and beyond.

Thank you, Bethany Davis, for your encouragement, honesty, and constructive editing. Editing science writing with a warm and loving eye is a gift.

Thank you, Dr. Alexe Bellingham, for your healing hands and your early support and enthusiasm for The Fascianation Method. You are a Godsend and undoubtedly helped drive our fascial care movement forward.

Thank you, Char Tarr, for showing up to our new class when no one else did, for allowing us to give you a new life, and for your immense generosity to help us travel for the cause.

Thank you to all of our clients and students. It's been a privilege to serve you all and hold your trust in our hands. We are grateful for your belief in us.

Thank you, Liana Mayo Kim, for your unceasing enthusiasm for this endeavor, for tapping into your energy reserves to lend your eagle eyes.

Thank you to The Paulos, The Chriscos, The Wilsons, The Torios, The Tibers, The Cuasito Clan, Channing Barringer, Ryan Andrews, Michael Peterson, Kirk Fritz, Bonnie Mahler, our compassionate Fascianation Method Trainers, and our Fascianator Production Crew. You have all made significant contributions to our optimism, sanity and beyond during the first tough years.

About the Authors

Eileen Paulo-Chrisco is the co-developer of The Fascianation Method for self-care, a founding member of the Fascia Research Society, and a 12 year fitness trainer 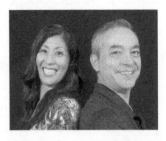 specializing in corrective exercise. Eileen thrives on helping people rediscover their abilities and joy by teaching them how to safely exercise and restore their body's ability to heal itself. Before becoming a Fascianation Method Practitioner, helping people with chronic pain and limited mobility, Eileen was a cell biologist and spent eighteen years as a biomedical and pharmaceutical researcher. She's a published author in the peer-reviewed scientific journal, *Cancer Research* and some of her work was utilized in research that was awarded the 2009 Nobel Prize for Physiology or Medicine. Eileen's career experience working with connective tissues and her nagging pains and discomforts led to a breakthrough. She realized that the limits of traditional Western medicine exist because connective tissue has not been recognized as an integral part of the immune system. She realized that healing chronic conditions causing discomfort or pain was very different from symptom management. Healing chronic health issues require a holistic care approach.

Anthony Chrisco has been called the Tony Robbins of fascia by many amongst his audience. Anthony's passion for transformation through fascial care is electric. Anthony is CEO of The Fascianator, a founding member of the Fascia Research Society, inventor of the Fascianator roller, the driver and leading developer of The Fascianation Method of self-myofascial release, a speaker, and a continuing education provider. With healing intuition, a love for movement science and 25 years of post-rehabilitation experience, he has joyfully helped people transcend physical limitations, chronic pain, and mental blocks by teaching people how to tune in and listen to what their body is saying. Anthony empowers other healers all around the globe by educating about human fascia and its implications in health and wellness. He was a member of the first Fascial Net Plastination Project in Germany, which would allow the world's first 3D exhibition of human fascia.

Eileen and Anthony travel globally to share their method of wellness, chronic pain relief, and body restoration. The Fascianation Method is received with tremendous success and offers incredible results in households, wellness studios, prestigious ballet companies, and its presence in educational and clinical institutions are on the rise! Eileen and Anthony reside with their two children, Channing and Malia, and their dog, Bruce. Although Bruce hasn't been trained to do self-myofascial release, the Chrisco family spoils him with daily myofascial massages.

Thank You!

Thank you for reading! We appreciate you, because you were receptive to the novel life changing healing concepts in our book. You took the time to learn more about the amazing human being that is waiting to be unleashed from the bondage of chronic pain!

If you enjoyed this book, a way to express your gratitude is to tell your friends and family about it and write a review so that others can be inspired to join the Fascial Care Movement!

It's one thing to read about The Fascianation Method and quite another to put it into action for frequent mind-body housekeeping. *We have a thank you present for you!*

Visit the website, painfreeeveryday.org, for:

- A free copy of The Fascianation Method Instructional E-Manual. The E-Manual has images that will help guide your body and Fascianator roller positioning to enable you to roll your pain away. Use it as a roadmap to take you on journey inside of your fascial organ system. You will visit your soft tissue restrictions, likely the root cause of your pain that today's routine diagnostic imaging tests do not detect.

- A discount coupon code for The Fascianator roller. You will not get the same results with just any body massage roller.

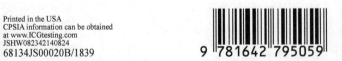